ABSOLUTE NUTRITION

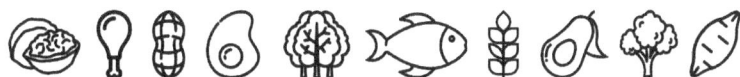

ABSOLUTE NUTRITION

THE COMPLETE GUIDE TO
NUTRITION & NUTRIENT-DENSE FOODS
AND MEALS FOR LIFELONG HEALTH

CHRISTOPHER D. SMITH

To all those aspiring to
a more nutritious diet and better health.

CONTENTS

Section I: Human Nutritional Evolution and How It Supports Our Health

Section II: Macronutrients

Section III: Micronutrients and Phytonutrients

Section IV: Nutrient-Dense and Nutritious Foods

Section V: Absolute Nutritious Meals

FOREWORD AND ACKNOWLEDGEMENTS

Does the world really need another book on diet and nutrition? That was the question I asked myself before starting this journey. Now, after two years of research and writing, the answer is a definitive *yes*.

There are thousands of studies and mountains of media content explaining diet and nutrition. The problem is that the information is just too much and, at the same time, not specific enough for regular people like you and me. This causes confusion and is a real barrier to building a practical diet full of the nutrition we need for good health.

There are many studies showing Americans believe their diets are healthy, when in fact they are not. One such study estimated that only 1% of Americans consume an "ideal" diet containing recommended levels of the most important food groups.[1] Many nutrition experts believe that we Americans simply do not understand what healthy eating looks like.

We shouldn't be all that surprised, given that:

- **Unhealthy foods dominate our supply chain:** Approximately 70% of the U.S. food supply is comprised of unhealthy, highly processed foods.[2]

- **The amount of information is overwhelming:** TV, books, and social media provide an avalanche of nutrition and food-related information and opinions. These are often confusing, contradictory, and misleading, or focus only on one food group or nutrient. As a result, many of us are constantly chasing the latest fad super foods or supplements, without achieving its promised health benefits.

- **Nutrition is complex:** There are approximately 40 essential nutrients that our bodies need from our daily diet. All of these nutrients are important for good health. Unless you are a nutritional scientist or dietician, you probably don't know the names of many of these. Even if you have heard of them, you may not know their specific health benefits, how much of each are needed, or the foods that provide them in healthy amounts.

What's missing is a simplified explanation of nutrition and dieting. That's what this book provides. It first gives you a basic description of nutrition and its health benefits.

Next, it identifies the most nutritious foods available in our local grocery stores. Lastly, it uses these foods to build examples of delicious affordable meals that contain recommended levels of the most important nutrients. With these meals as your guide, you will be able to build your own healthy diet. If you regularly consume these meals, then you will achieve absolute nutrition with daily recommended levels of almost all essential nutrients.

I have a unique perspective from that of the physicians, scientists, and dieticians who typically write books in this space. Like you, I used to build my meals based on suggestions from TV shows, internet articles, and social media. I thought I was eating a fully healthy diet. In truth, I wasn't. Now I am, and if you read this book and follow its recommendations, you will too.

My Approach to This Book

I have spent the last two years reviewing all the diet and nutrition information sources I could find on the internet. I synthesized this information and translated it into succinct, straightforward recommendations, creating a specific guide for building a healthy diet and preparing nutritious meals.

My research and recommendations relied on only the most credible information sources. I reviewed dozens of studies published by the National Institutes of Health (NIH), the U.S. government's primary agency for biomedical and public health research, and the *Journal of the American Medical Association* (JAMA), a leading peer-reviewed medical journal published by the American Medical Association. I also read hundreds of articles from nationally recognized health associations, government websites, and respected online journals, including The American Heart Association, American Diabetes Association, American Cancer Society, Centers for Disease Control and Prevention (CDC), Academy of Nutrition and Dietetics, and American Society for Nutrition, among others. Lastly, I reviewed the websites of several highly respected academic medical centers and health publications. These sources are cited throughout, with full bibliographic information included at the end of the book. These citations include the URL link for these sources in case you are interested in greater detail.

In addition, I used the USDA's FoodData Central website for analyzing and identifying the most nutritious foods. It is considered one of the most credible food nutritional data sources in the world.

Lastly, I had a highly credentialled dietician review key parts of the book, and she endorsed my food and meal recommendations. All these steps helped ensure that the information provided in this book follows, when available, the best advice of many of the leading minds and organizations in the science of nutrition and food.

In the course of my research, I also found that while many experts recommend eating a "well-balanced diet," and certain food groups, none clearly explain the exact foods to eat, their precise nutrient levels, or how to build highly nutritious meals using those foods. This critical information is missing not only from the resources listed above but also from many respected dietary plans. This book aims to fill that gap.

My Diet and Nutrition Story

Why do I care so much about diet and nutrition that I was willing to write an entire book on it? First, I have the same goal as you: a long and healthy life.

Second, I have always been keenly interested in health and wellness. This goes back to my childhood, when several of my relatives passed away early in life. My maternal grandfather died in his early 50s. My other grandfather and both grandmothers had all passed by age 70, and several other relatives also passed away relatively early in life, mostly men. Cardiovascular issues, like heart attack and stroke, and cancer were the main causes.

These deaths occurred when I was young, and they made a significant impression on me. My mother often warned me that we had "bad genes," so I better take care of myself. I literally thought I would be lucky to make it to age 60. I therefore embraced a healthy diet and exercise early in life.

Thanks to My Friends and Family

Writing this book was a long journey, and I was lucky to have many people support me throughout it. The first person I want to thank is my good friend Jim, who is like a big brother to me. Jim has written several very successful books and was willing to share his insights into the process during our monthly dinners at our favorite Mexican restaurant. I couldn't have done it without you and your encouragement, brother.

Several people also supported me by providing feedback on initial drafts of the book. I want to thank one of my very best friends, Greg. He took the time to read through many preliminary sections of the book and was always brutally honest about what needed improvement. I winced a little at some of his comments, but he was right and I needed to hear them. I will always be grateful for his help and friendship.

Two other long-time friends were also supportive reviewers. Laurie and Kary were the most committed in terms of evaluating the manuscript and encouraging me to write the book. Both were timely and detailed with their feedback, helpfully identifying critical areas where the book needed more information and where it needed less. This book is much easier to read because of them.

Another early reader was my friend Hooman. The best physical therapist in Atlanta, he is well trained and educated in many areas of health and wellness. We discussed the book often when he was helping me recover from a torn ACL. His knowledge and feedback were critical in improving the early drafts.

I also must thank Sydney Flippo, a very talented and knowledgeable dietician in Los Angeles and a fellow Virginia Tech Hokie. She reviewed several sections of the book, provided insightful feedback, and assured me that I was on the right track with my recommended foods and meals.

It wouldn't be right to leave out some dear friends that patiently listened to me over the last two years as I incessantly talked about the book and nutrition. Lane and Stephanie heard more than their fair share about nutrition and different foods during our travels and over many dinners. They were always gracious listeners and at least seemingly interested, asking insightful questions.

Also, my great friend Todd heard all about the book during our many hikes. As always, he was a great listener and very enthusiastic. Having these good friends to talk to helped me solidify my thoughts and articulate my positions on key points.

Lastly, I want to thank my two children, Garrett and Cate. Post-college, they both lived with me for several months while I was writing the book. They were patient with me in the mornings, letting their dad be glued to his computer reading articles and typing away. I love you both very much. Also, Garrett's girlfriend Phoebe was always so positive and interested when I discussed the book. She is a dear.

I'm very blessed to have all these people in my life and am thankful for their friendship, love, and incredible support.

INTRODUCTION

I think we all can agree that we'd like to live a long life. Surveys show most of us want to live into our 80s and many want to reach 100 years of age, but with one big caveat: We only want such longevity if we're healthy.[3, 4]

What if I told you I have one simple strategy that greatly increases your chances of leading a long and healthy life? There are a lot of lifestyle behaviors that can help, but one of the most important is a healthy diet, one that provides us with all the nutrients our bodies need for good health.

You may be thinking you already know this, but do you really know what a healthy diet looks like? A recent survey found that over 70% of Americans rate their diets as healthy. This same survey had nutritional experts assess the diets of the survey respondents. Almost all earned a "D" or "F" grade, in other words poor and needing significant improvement.[5]

The average American now consumes over half their daily calories from highly processed foods (also known as ultra-processed foods). Even more disturbing, two-thirds of our children's calories come from these foods.[6]

These foods often strip out natural nutrients during processing and contain unhealthily high levels of other ingredients. The result is that most of us don't take in adequate levels of the most important nutrients, and consume unnaturally high levels of added sugar, sodium, saturated fats, and calories. This is causing a severe health crisis.

🔍 Did You Know (DYK)

The average U.S. adult consumes 17 teaspoons of added sugar every day. That adds up to 130 cups of added sugar per year, or over 60 pounds! The result of this dietary habit is over 100,000 extra calories or potentially 40 pounds of added weight annually![7]

A diet regularly full of highly processed foods will greatly lower the chances of a long and healthy life. Further, these foods often make us very sick long before we ever reach old age. Countless studies show that these foods are a primary cause of chronic conditions like cancer, cardiovascular disease, diabetes, obesity, high blood pressure, kidney disease, Alzheimer's, arthritis, osteoporosis, and mental illness.

Six in ten U.S. adults now have at least one chronic condition, and over 40% have two or more. Eight of the ten leading causes of U.S. deaths are from one of these conditions. Children are also contracting them at unprecedented levels.

These foods are costing us our health and negatively impacting our healthcare system. Over 90% of all U.S. healthcare dollars are now spent treating chronic conditions.[8] [9]

Even if you are not eating a lot of highly processed foods, there's a good chance you are falling short of the daily recommendations for several important nutrients. These nutrient inadequacies are also a major cause of chronic conditions.

If you are waiting for our healthcare system to fix this crisis, don't hold your breath. The U.S. healthcare industry's "fee for service" financial model is built on treating these conditions, not preventing them. The industry gets paid every time a patient is seen and treated by a healthcare provider.

Given this model, there are few financial incentives to prevent or even reduce the prevalence of these conditions. Doing so would erode the industry's primary source of revenue. The U.S. government has been unsuccessful thus far in addressing this issue.

This is a sobering situation, but there is hope. It is within our control to do something to help prevent these conditions, and one thing we can all do is eat a fully nutritious diet. In this book, I'm going to show you how to build the diet you need for good health and longevity.

The Solution

Over 2,000 years ago, the Greek philosopher Hippocrates stated, "let food be thy medicine and medicine be thy food." Hippocrates is considered the father of medicine, and he nailed this advice.

When regularly eating a variety of the healthiest foods, we give our bodies the essential nutrients they need to perform as intended. We're talking about normal brain function, healthy heartbeat and blood flow, high energy levels, strong muscles, sturdy bones, and a powerful immune system that protects us from all types of diseases. Without these nutrients, our bodies struggle with these important functions.

Developing meals complete with all essential nutrients sounds simple, but it is not. The truth is that understanding nutrition and building a healthy diet is difficult. It requires knowing the nutrient content of all our potential foods, selecting the most nutritious ones, and then building a daily meal plan around those foods. This is complicated stuff!

Most of us don't have the time to educate ourselves to this level or to put in the effort to develop such a diet. We have busy lives and other priorities.

Often, we struggle to build such a diet and instead turn to fad food groups, or single nutrient supplements, or rely on "magic" pills to cure our health issues and help us lose weight. Television, social media, and the internet all encourage us to buy these products and erroneously promise them as silver-bullet solutions.

I know, as I used to get my diet and nutritional informa-tion from these same sources. As a result, my diet became a hodgepodge of different recommended foods and supple-ments. I now know this approach left me with a diet well below recommended levels for several important nutrients.

Even well-known diet plans can confuse us into making poor nutrition decisions. Most are simply not specific enough about the nutrients to target, or the foods, serving sizes, and meals that will ensure your diet is truly healthy and contains the absolute nutrition your body needs.

The good news: This book has done all the hard work for you. It provides you with everything you need to know to build a fully nutritious diet. Here is what you can expect:

Section I describes the evolution of human nutrition and how our bodies' systems use nutrition to maintain good health. These include our digestive gut microbiota, metabolisms, and immune systems. If you have ever wanted to know more about these health areas (and oxidative stress and antioxidants), these chapters provide a good summary.

Section II explains the details of each type of macronutrient, their importance to our health, and the daily amounts we should be getting. It includes descriptions of proteins, fats, and carbohydrates, and summarizes macronutrient subcategories like fiber and omega-3s. This section further recommends limits on saturated fats and added sugar.

Section III focuses primarily on micronutrients. It identifies the most important micronutrients for good health and describes the ones most Americans struggle to consume at adequate levels. I also include a brief section on phytonutrients. While the science around phytonutrients is still developing, studies show they have potentially significant health benefits. Examples of these include beta-carotene and resveratrol.

Section IV identifies many of the most nutritious animal and plant foods available in the U.S. You will likely be familiar with most, if not all, of these foods. The descriptions will help you better understand their nutrient values. This section also includes a list of my top 10 nutrient-dense foods as well as some honorable mentions. If you include these top foods regularly in your diet, then you are well on your way towards getting the absolute nutrition you need for good health.

Section V goes a step further by utilizing these foods to develop highly nutritious meals. This gives you a jump start on building your own healthy diet. For each meal, I evaluate its nutrients compared to daily recommended levels and suggest methods to enhance the meal's nutritional value. Most of these meals cost well under $10 per serving.

The foods I focus on are not exotic or expensive. They are all sitting in your local grocery store waiting for you. You just need to know which foods are nutrient-dense, select them, and eat them regularly.

Armed with this information, my hope is that you will be inspired to incorporate these foods and meals into your diet. After all, you want to have a long healthy life, right? If this is your goal, this book will help you achieve it.

I am living proof of this fact. My research for the book has resulted in me changing my diet. I now consume nutrient-dense foods with more protein, healthy carbohydrates, fiber, and unsaturated fats. My meals provide me with the daily recommended levels of nearly all vitamins and minerals. They also contain only healthy levels of sugar, sodium, and saturated fats.

These changes to my diet have helped increase my energy levels, maintain a healthy weight, and keep my blood panel health measures within normal ranges. I also believe my overall sense of wellbeing and mood have improved. I have no chronic conditions and take no medications for my health. At 62, I'm happy with these results, especially given my family history of chronic illness and early death.

I cannot guarantee you will achieve the same results, but there is a mountain of evidence that shows a nutritious diet will greatly improve your chances of longevity and good health.

How My Nutrient-Dense Diet Compares to Other Diets

Several well-known diets focus on individual macronutrients. Some restrict fat intake as a primary goal, for example, while others restrict carbohydrate intake, and still others make high protein intake the primary goal. Some diets use a combination of these goals.

From my research, these diets may be helpful with short-term weight loss but often are not sustainable. Further, some of these diets may increase your risk of other health problems.

For example, a high protein/low carb diet would typically be high in animal foods, and lower in plant foods and dairy. The problem is that plant foods contain many important macronutrients, micronutrients, and phytonutrients that are difficult, if not impossible, to get at adequate levels from animal foods. Missing out on these key nutrients is not healthy for you. Further, this same diet may allow you to select meats high in saturated fats, which may increase your risk of cardiovascular disease.

Other diets recommend balancing macronutrients and focusing on certain food groups. This is more consistent with the recommendations in this book. The Mediterranean and DASH diets are both popular diets that focus on whole plant-based foods for healthy carbohydrates and fats. For protein, the Mediterranean diet emphasizes fish, while the DASH diet focuses more on lean cuts of meat and low-fat dairy.

Overall, these two are very good diet plans and certainly much healthier than most Americans' current diets. However, I believe my nutrient dense-foods approach has advantages over both these diets.

1. **It focuses on specific foods, not food groups.** My approach concentrates on highly nutritious foods, while

both the Mediterranean and DASH diets focus more on food groups. Not all foods within a food group are created nutritionally equal.

For example, both diets promote whole grains, which I agree with. However, there is a big difference between whole-wheat bread and corn. 100% whole-wheat bread is a nutrient-dense food. A serving size of two slices has moderate to high levels of nearly all B vitamins, vitamin E, and all priority minerals. It also has moderate levels of protein, polyunsaturated fats, and fiber. A serving size of corn (one ear) contains moderate levels of three B vitamins but is low in protein, unsaturated fats, fiber, and all priority minerals. While corn contains several nutrients, it is not nutrient-dense food like whole-wheat bread.

2. **It defines specific serving sizes.** A food's nutrient levels depend on its nutrient density and the serving size consumed. The Mediterranean diet does not state specific serving sizes for its food groups. The DASH diet does give example serving sizes, but not specific serving sizes for all foods. In addition, several of these example serving sizes are not consistent with typical serving sizes in the U.S. This lack of specificity on food quantity can make a big difference.

As an example, a single-cup serving of blackberries provides high levels of vitamins C and K as well as fiber. It also has moderate amounts of vitamin E, iron, and omega-3 ALA. If you eat just a quarter cup, you are only getting moderate amounts of vitamin C. It is low in omega-3 ALA, vitamins K and E, iron, and fiber.

3. **It identifies priority nutrients**. The Mediterranean diet focuses on certain food groups, not specific nutrients. The DASH diet focuses on a few nutrients (calcium, potassium, magnesium, fiber, and protein) but ignores several other very important ones. Those missing include omega-3s, omega-6, monounsaturated fats, all vitamins, choline, and the minerals zinc and iron. These are incredibly important nutrients for good health. My diet approach ensures you get these!

We Can All Do This!

I realize it's challenging to change your diet. Whatever your current meal habits, you probably like the foods and meals you eat. Change may not be easy.

If you regularly eat highly processed foods, this will mean significantly changing your diet. I hope as you read the book, you begin to realize how critical nutrition is to your and your family's good health. Also, as you review the example meals I've developed, you may be surprised to find that most will be very familiar to you. There's a good chance you grew up eating many of them.

If you feel you already have a healthy diet, this transition will likely be easier. You are probably already eating many of my recommended foods, and while the food serving sizes and combinations in my meal examples may be new, the meals them-selves will be familiar. I also believe you will find these meals to be delicious and easy to prepare.

You may be questioning the costs of these meals, and you need not worry. Most of my meal examples cost $5–10 per serving. If they cost more, I recommend alternatives that reduce the cost.

To support your changing eating habits, I have highlighted the most nutritious foods available throughout the book. There may be some repetition, but I think this will help you better understand and remember them. In addition, in the last section of the book (Section V) I recommend several specific diet and meal strategies that should make the transition easier.

Approaches for Reading the Book

I realize interests concerning food, nutrition, and diet vary. Some of you may be nutritional junkies (like me). You want to know the "why" to this dietary approach. Others of you may not care about the why; you just want to know what foods to eat and how to incorporate them into your meals.

This book is structured to satisfy the needs of both types of readers. If you fit into the "why" camp, you will want to read the whole book. This approach provides you with a great overview of nutrition and explains many critical nutrients you may have heard about but may not clearly understand from a health perspective.

If you do not care about the "why" and just want to know what to eat and how to combine these into meals, you can skip to Sections IV and V. This approach reduces the reading time but still provides an education on nutritious foods and meals that will help you build a healthy diet.

As you read, you will see key facts and dietary strategies labeled *Did You Know (DYK)* and *Pro Move* placed in reading boxes. The DYK call-outs provide a quick fact relating to the particular topic being discussed. The Pro Move call-outs suggest how to take your nutrients or foods to an even higher level. I have included these elements for those interested in more information, but they are not critical for understanding the topic.

I've also added a few short *Facts Break* call-outs. Their purpose is to provide relief from all the details in these sections, providing a pause at times when your brain may be hurting. As with the DYK and Pro Move call-outs, these are not necessary for understanding the information. Feel free to skip them if you are not interested. For those so inclined, enjoy!

I hope you enjoy the book and get a lot out of it. My overall wish is for you to find at least some aspects that inspire you to improve your diet. Best of luck with your journey!

Additional sources used for Introduction: [10] [11] [12] [13]

SECTION I

Human Nutritional Evolution and How It Supports Our Health

This section is a simplified explanation of how we humans evolved to eat a natural diet full of fresh meats and whole plant foods (Chapter 1). It also summarizes the science of how our bodies digest and extract nutrients and the health significance of our gut microbiota (Chapter 2). Next, it explains the role our metabolisms play in producing and using needed proteins, fatty acids, glucose, and micronutrients for key bodily functions (Chapter 3).

Finally, the section discusses how nutrients support our immune systems in protecting us from diseases and toxins and the potential health implications for metabolic syndrome and obesity (Chapter 4).

With this information, you will have a good, basic under-standing of why and how our bodies need nutrition and its importance to our health. It provides a great background for the next two sections that describe the most important nutrients in our foods: macronutrients, micronutrients, and phytonutrients.

Before moving on to Chapter 1, I'd like to begin with where nutrients come from. This will help you better understand how humans evolved to use these nutrients for good health.

How do nutrients get into our foods? The simple answer is that they come from the many natural elements found in Earth's land, water, and atmosphere. They provide all the elements required for life: oxygen, carbon, hydrogen, nitrogen, and many more (remember the periodic table?). All the foods and nutrients we consume contain some combination of these elements.

This is where plants come in. It's believed that plant life on Earth's land masses developed approximately 500 million years ago. Plants use the elements and sun to make their own food and nutrients. During photosynthesis, plants produce oxygen as well as proteins, fats, carbohydrates, and vitamins. Plants further absorb and use minerals from the soil via their roots. They store excess nutrients in their leaves, stems, roots, fruits, and seeds.

Why the botany lesson? Because without plants, animal life is impossible. Plants provide us with oxygen to breathe and also give us, directly or indirectly, all essential nutrients. This includes important macronutrients, micronutrients, phytonutri-ents, and fiber.

Now that we've answered the question of where nutrients come from, let's move on to a brief history of human nutrition. This provides context for today's nutritional environment, which is very different from the one humans had for most of our existence.

CHAPTER 1

Our Nutritional Evolution

The human body and its complex systems were formed through evolution. It is believed that the first humans came into existence approximately 300,000 years ago, evolving from our human-like ancestors, called hominins. Our evolution continues today as we adapt to the ever-changing conditions on Earth.

To understand how humans evolved from a nutritional perspective, it's helpful to appreciate three unique time periods that defined human lifestyle and food consumption. These are known as the hunter-gatherer, agricultural, and industrial/modern periods.[14] [15]

Hunter-gatherer period: This period lasted from humanity's beginnings until approximately 12,000 years ago. It is known as the Pleistocene period and represents over 96% of human existence.

During this period, humans were food generalists, consuming large varieties of wild plants and animal foods. Their diet was likely seasonal, meaning they ate whatever edible plants and animals were available during certain periods of the year. It is believed their diet was approximately 80% plants and 20% animals, but environmental factors in different parts of the world likely greatly impacted these percentages.

The hunter-gatherers are believed to have consumed a much broader diet of plants and animals than in later human periods. Their whole plant foods were high in complex carbohydrates, unsaturated fats, vitamins, minerals, and fiber. Wild animal foods provided lean proteins with healthy levels of saturated and unsaturated fats, and many vitamins and minerals. As with wild game today, the animals hunter-gatherers consumed were likely lower in saturated fat than modern domesticated animals.

Over time, the growing human brain and body size required more protein. This resulted in an increased consumption of animal foods. Also, cooking of foods began in this period, helping to enhance the absorption of nutrients and improving the taste of the food.

The hunter-gatherer's diet and lifestyle were overall very healthy for their environment. These early humans relied on their food to provide them with the adaptability needed to migrate and survive throughout the world. Their constant physical activity and diverse diet of fresh meats and whole plant foods were perfectly suited for human energy and nutritional needs. Evolution made sure of it.

Based on studies of early human bones and teeth, it appears that the non-communicable diseases (chronic diseases) of today were virtually non-existent and communicable diseases (infectious diseases) very limited. This last health issue was likely, at least in part, due to the relatively low population density of humans at the time.

This is not to insinuate the hunter-gather life was utopian. It is believed that infant mortality was very high compared to more recent times. These humans also encountered survival challenges from wild animals, periods of food scarcity, and less protection from environmental elements.

Agricultural period: This period began around 12,000 years ago, after the last ice age, and lasted until approximately 250 years ago. Humans began transitioning into settlements with crop cultivation and domesticating animals for reliable food sources. Most of this time is known as the Neolithic period and it represents approximately 4% of human existence.

Over time, high-yield crops such as grains and legumes, and other plant foods like carrots, lettuce, and certain herbs, became agricultural staples. Dried grains and legumes were perfect for storing to help meet future food needs. Some wild plants continued to be used as a food source.

Cattle, sheep, goats, and pigs were the primary animals raised for food. At the start of this period, it is estimated that plant foods comprised approximately 75% of the diet, while animal foods made up about 25%, although this likely varied by region.

With consistently available food sources, this period offered humans some independence from nature and its volatile cycles. As a result, Earth's human population grew significantly.

Human health was mixed during this period. Communicable diseases increased with population growth. It was also common for domesticated animals to live in close quarters with humans. This caused unsanitary conditions and a breeding ground for insects. Communicable diseases from this period are still evident today, including cholera, tuberculosis, plague, hepatitis B, smallpox, measles, malaria, typhus, brucellosis, and salmonella.

Compared to the hunter-gatherers, these humans were less active and ate a less balanced diet. This resulted in the first occurrence of some noncommunicable diseases and some of these exist today as chronic conditions.

Industrial revolution/modern period: This period began approximately 250 years ago and continues today. It represents less than one-tenth of 1% of human existence. In it, we humans continue to manipulate our environment and change our food-consumption patterns and lifestyles.

Starting in the second half of the eighteenth century, the industrial revolution produced advancements in machines which reduced the need for farm workers and created factory jobs. This resulted in many people transitioning from the countryside to cities to work in factories.

To feed these large and growing city populations, new food processing and preservation techniques emerged, such as canning. These processed foods had a longer shelf life and were easier to stockpile. They were also cheaper and immediately ready for everyday consumption. Unfortunately, these highly processed foods were lower in nutrients and included many chemicals.

The consumption of highly processed foods continues today and has accelerated. To feed an expanding world population and improve taste (and profits), current industrial food processes with milling and high heating often eliminate or greatly reduce the natural nutritional elements in plant foods. For animal foods, less natural diets and poor living conditions can increase animal size and yield but result in less healthy nutrients. These foods often contain unnaturally high levels of certain ingredients, such as added sugar, added sodium, and saturated fat. Further, many are unnaturally high in calories.

Americans today consume more than half our daily calories from these foods. As mentioned in the foreword, over 70% of all foods available to Americans are highly processed. They are not just in fast food restaurants; these foods also dominate the shelves of our grocery stores.

When added to our increasingly sedentary lifestyles, the health consequences are catastrophic. Diets full of these foods have resulted in chronic diseases reaching pandemic levels.

Why are these foods so unhealthy for modern humans? Because for more than 99% of our evolution, they did not exist. Our bodies evolved primarily during the hunter-gatherer period, adapted to a diet full of natural foods rich in lean proteins, complex carbohydrates, healthy fats, vitamins, minerals, phyto-nutrients, and fiber. None of these foods were naturally high in sodium, and there was no such thing as added sugar.

Our bodies' systems are built for the hunter-gatherer diet, not for the highly processed foods of today. Human biological evolution has struggled to keep up with these changes to our diet, and our health has suffered as a result.

Let's now dive into how some of the body's most important systems use nutrition for good health and explore the negative health consequences of highly processed foods.

CHAPTER 2

How Our Bodies Use Nutrition: Digestive System

W hen we think of our bodies, we tend to focus on the physical components such as our brains, skin, bones, muscles, organ systems, blood, etc. However, the body also has several important support systems that allow these physical components to work effectively and maintain good health. These systems perform their functions at a microscopic level.

The systems I am referring to are our digestive tracts, gut microbiota, metabolisms, and immune systems. When performing normally, these systems effectively produce energy; promote brain health; support strong bones and muscles; maintain healthy blood levels of glucose, cholesterol, fats, and oxygen; and protect us from harmful microorganisms, toxins, and other body stressors.

In this chapter, I focus on how our digestive systems help absorb nutrients from our foods, and the health importance of our gut microbiota.

Digestive System

This seems like a logical place to start a book on nutrition! The digestive system processes all the foods and liquids ingested. This system includes the mouth, esophagus, stomach, small intestine, and large intestine. The digestive tract's purpose is to extract key nutrients and separate out non-digestible material for waste elimination. The liver, pancreas, and gallbladder are organs that support the digestive process.

DYK

The average person consumes approximately 60 tons of food and 15–20,000 gallons of liquids over their lifetime. Our digestive systems process every scrap and drop!

During digestion, foods are broken down into smaller particles that allow valuable nutrients to be extracted for use. These nutrients include proteins, fats, carbohydrates, fiber, vitamins, and minerals. The small intestine finalizes this breakdown using enzymes and absorbs these nutrients into the bloodstream. Most are then delivered to the liver.

The liver is a critical organ, as it filters and regulates our blood to ensure these nutrients are in the correct chemical form for use by the body and are maintained at healthy levels. It also stores some nutrients for future use and delivers these into the bloodstream as needed.

Gut Microbiota

The digestive tract is greatly supported by trillions of microorganisms, including bacteria, fungi, and viruses. These microorganisms live in the digestive tract and are called the gut microbiota. Most are in the large intestine.

A healthy microbiota supports metabolic functions, synthesis of certain vitamins, and some nutrient absorption. It also communicates with the brain through neurotransmitters and hormones to influence immune system and gut responses. This is the so-called "gut-brain axis."

Studies show that a healthy microbiota has a stable, diverse, and high number of "good" microorganisms. Our diets have a significant impact on our microbiota. A key step for building and maintaining a healthy microbiota is to consume a diverse diet full of whole plant foods and fermented foods that contain prebiotics and probiotics.

Prebiotics are the fiber and certain starches in plant foods. They are found in vegetables, fruits, whole grains, nuts, legumes, and seeds. Prebiotics help to feed and nourish healthy microbiota organisms. Unfortunately, most Americans consume far too little fiber and starch.

Probiotics are food groups that add their own healthy microorganisms to our microbiota. Fermented foods such as sauerkraut, kefir, kimchi, yogurt, and miso are good examples. Probiotics help to add microorganism diversity to the microbiota.

An unhealthy microbiota can result in metabolic issues that increase the risk of infections, obesity, type 2 diabetes, inflammation, allergies, and digestive disorders. In addition, studies show an unhealthy microbiota can negatively affect mental health and increase the risk of cardiovascular disease and some cancers.

Other studies have shown that certain food types are destructive to our microbiota diversity. These include foods high in refined sugar, high-fructose corn syrup, artificial sweeteners, and sodium, as well as fried foods cooked in oils high in saturated fats. Smoking, excess alcohol consumption, stress, lack of sleep, depression, and frequently taking antibiotics can also negatively impact our microbiota.

📖 Digestive System Facts Break

➜ The digestive system tract is approximately 30 feet long, with the small intestine alone measuring over 20 feet.

➜ The mouth produces over two pints of saliva per day.

➜ The time from eating food to elimination varies by person and generally takes 14 hours to 2 1/2 days.

➜ The average stomach can handle four pounds of food at one time.

➜ Flatulence (passing gas) is caused by bacteria in the digestive tract. The average person passes gas 13–21 times per day!

Additional sources used for gut microbiota description: [16] [17] [18]

CHAPTER 3

How Our Bodies Use Nutrition: Metabolism of Proteins, Fats, Carbohydrates, and Micronutrients

B efore writing this book, my limited understanding of metabolism was that if it's fast, you don't gain weight. Well, it turns out that's not exactly the case. In fact, studies show that many obese people have higher metabolisms than the non-obese.

The real purpose of metabolism is to perform trillions of daily chemical reactions that support many body functions. One of the most important roles of the metabolism is to assist the digestive tract in breaking down food into more usable forms. It helps extract nutrients out of this food so that they can then be used to support several bodily functions.

Proteins and Amino Acids

Proteins are molecules made up of smaller particles called amino acids. The body makes many of its own proteins, but it needs help making others. This help comes from the proteins and amino acids contained in our foods.

During digestion, metabolic chemical reactions draw the proteins out of food and break them down into different amino acids. These amino acids are then absorbed into the bloodstream and transferred to the liver. The liver then either releases them to cells to make new proteins or uses them directly to create other new proteins.

These newly created proteins are in a form that the body and its cells can use for key functions. One of the primary functions of proteins is to support cell structure growth, maintenance, and repair. These structures include cells in our muscles, bones, brains, organs, and skin.

Other new proteins support metabolic reactions for maintaining pH balance, strengthening the immune system and transporting and storing nutrients in the body.

There are nine essential amino acids from dietary proteins used to make new proteins. Animal food proteins contain all nine of these amino acids, but most plant foods have only some. The good news is we can get all nine by eating a variety of plant foods.

In Section II, I recommend much higher levels of daily protein than the current U.S. recommendations. This is especially needed for active people. If these higher levels were applied to the average U.S. adult, most of us would not meet this recommended level.

Weight management and weight loss can also be helped by consuming higher levels of protein. Studies have shown that protein consumption increases satiety (feeling full) and maintains higher muscle mass, which burns more calories.

Fats and Fatty Acids

Digested fats include saturated, polyunsaturated, and monounsaturated. These fats are broken down into fatty acids during digestion. In the small intestine, fatty acids are metabolized into blood lipids called triglycerides and transported into the bloodstream.

Triglycerides are used by the body's cells for energy; those not used are stored in fat cells called adipocytes. The body draws on these stored triglycerides for future energy needs. This energy source is mostly used to fuel low-to-medium intensity activities, long endurance exercise, and normal metabolic functions. Fats in foods are the most energy dense of all macronutrients and contain nine calories per gram (protein and carbohydrates have only four calories per gram).

DYK

The number of adipocyte cells (fat cells) is determined by late adolescence and rarely changes during adulthood. Fat cells increase or decrease in size (and drive our weight up or down) depending on the number of triglycerides stored or used.

Another well-known blood lipid is **cholesterol**. Primarily produced by the liver, its purpose is to maintain cell membranes and produce essential hormones. Cholesterol comes in two forms of lipids, low-density lipoproteins (LDL) and high-density lipoproteins (HDL). Both LDL ("bad" cholesterol) and HDL ("good" cholesterol) are needed for healthy body function.

The liver regulates the amount of cholesterol in the bloodstream by producing it or eliminating excess amounts depending on the body's needs. It is thought that when there are large amounts of LDL in the bloodstream, the liver can become overwhelmed and not eliminate this excess entirely. This leads to high levels of bloodstream LDL. High blood levels of LDL and triglycerides are associated with several health issues and these are described in detail in Section 2, Chapter 6.

Carbohydrates and Glucose

Whole plant foods have what are called complex and simple carbohydrates, which contain sugars. When these sugars are digested, they produce glucose. Glucose is the main energy source used by the body. Once digested, this glucose is transferred into the bloodstream and either delivered to cells for energy use or stored in the liver for future energy needs.

Glucose is the energy source we use when we are active. Our muscles, immune systems, and brains use glucose heavily and need it to function properly.

The liver is the principal organ that regulates blood glucose levels. It does this by metabolizing excess glucose into glycogen, which it then stores. When more energy is needed, the liver transforms this glycogen back into glucose and releases it into the bloodstream.

When glucose enters the bloodstream, the pancreas releases a hormone called insulin. Insulin allows glucose to enter cells for energy use.

DYK

Glucose is metabolized in our cells into a molecule called adenosine triphosphate (ATP) so that it can then be used for energy.

Metabolism Facts Break

→ *Our bodies' cells are constantly undergoing metabolic reactions. During overnight sleep, our metabolisms typically burn 300–400 calories.*

→ *Daily habits can greatly affect the rate of our metabolisms.*

→ *Muscle growth increases metabolism and burns more calories than fat. Build those muscles!*

→ *High-intensity exercise is believed to rev up our metabolisms, even up to several hours later.*

→ *Skipping meals, calorie restrictive diets, and fasting can all slow down metabolism.*

→ *Poor sleep quality can also slow metabolism.*

Additional sources used for the protein, fats, carbohydrates, and metabolism descriptions: [19] [20] [21] [22] [23] [24] [25]

Micronutrients—Vitamins and Minerals

Consuming foods with healthy levels of vitamins and minerals is critical for good health. Our metabolisms support the absorption of micronutrients. In turn, these nutrients work with our metabolisms to provide our cells with energy and oxygen; support cell development, growth, and function; and help our bodies protect themselves from a condition called oxidative stress.

Energy is constantly needed by our bodies to function properly. As described above, this energy comes primarily from carbohydrates in the form of glucose, but also from fats and, in some instances, proteins. While our muscles and brains use much of this energy, all the body's systems need it throughout the day, even when at rest.

Certain micronutrients are key for metabolic energy production from proteins, fats, and carbohydrates. These nutrients support the creation of enzymes that extract amino acids, triglycerides, and glucose. The micronutrients most involved in energy production include most B vitamins, vitamin C, magnesium, and iron.

DYK

The adult human brain is only 2% of our body weight but consumes approximately 20% of the body's energy and 20% of its oxygen. This supports the brain's constant activity, even during sleep. [26][27]

Oxygen is needed by the body's cells to use energy. The lungs and respiratory system take in oxygen and transfer it into the bloodstream. The cardiovascular system transports this oxygen via red blood cells to all cell locations within the body.

With the support of certain micronutrients, the metabolism's role is to get the oxygen into these red blood cells via hemoglobin. Our metabolisms also help transfer this oxygen into our cells. Iron and several B vitamins are essential to the formation of hemoglobin and red blood cells.

Inadequate intake of iron and vitamins B9 and B12 can cause **anemia,** a low level of healthy red blood cells with hemoglobin. Anemia can affect mental focus, muscle performance, and stamina.

Cell development and function are also supported by metabolic functions with the help of micronutrients. Our metabolisms support the formation and growth of healthy cells throughout the body and their function. This support includes producing brain cells, forming neurotransmitters, and supporting nerve transmissions. Several B vitamins, vitamin C, magnesium, and iron are all important to these metabolic functions. Calcium, potassium, and zinc are particularly important in supporting brain function.

Oxidative stress occurs when free radicals overwhelm our bodies' defenses against them. Free radicals are naturally occurring molecules that form during normal metabolic functions (e.g., digestion, energy use during exercise, etc.). Free radicals can also result from external sources of stress, such as excessive alcohol consumption, smoking, radiation, pollution, and some medicines. Illness, injury, stress, and poor sleep are also thought to contribute to the formation of free radicals.

There is complicated chemistry involved with their formation, but the key point is that too many free radicals can cause oxidative stress. This condition can alter cell DNA, proteins, carbohydrates, and fats (lipids). These alterations can damage or even kill cells and impair macronutrient use, which can harm key organs and increase inflammation.

Studies show that, over time, unregulated oxidative stress can contribute to the development of several chronic conditions, including cancer, cardiovascular disease, neurological diseases (Alzheimer's and Parkinson's), diabetes, kidney disease, arthritis, osteoporosis, sarcopenia, and metabolic syndrome.

So, how do we mitigate the effects of free radicals? Our bodies have natural defenses against them, called antioxidants. **Antioxidants** offset free radicals by reducing their effects or rendering them harmless. For example, glutathione is a strong antioxidant naturally produced by the body to defend against free radicals.

We also get antioxidants from our food. Vitamins A, C, D, E, and several Bs are all considered antioxidants or have anti-oxidant properties. In addition, the minerals zinc, magnesium, selenium, and copper have antioxidant properties. There are many credible studies showing that consuming foods high in anti-oxidants is important for reducing the effects of oxidative stress.

In addition, many plant foods have what are called phyto-nutrients, which also have antioxidant properties. These phytonutrients include carotenoids with beta-carotene, flavonoids, organosulfur compounds, phenolic acids and phytoestrogens.

Lastly, we can protect our bodies from free radicals by avoiding or reducing some of the stressors listed above (e.g., smoking, etc.).

The bottom line is that we can help our bodies get energy and oxygen and increase our natural defenses against oxidative stress by regularly consuming a variety of foods high in micro-nutrients and phytonutrients.

Section III will describe in detail the most important micro-nutrients and phytonutrients to help support your body and promote good health.

Additional sources used for micronutrients, energy, oxygen, and oxidative stress descriptions: [28] [29] [30] [31] [32] [33]

CHAPTER 4

The Immune System and Metabolic Syndrome

mmune health and a condition called metabolic syndrome are two areas significantly impacted by poor nutrition. Many U.S. adults struggle with these health areas. I highlight these here because I believe that several recommendations in this book could help reduce the frequency and severity of these and related health conditions.

Immune System

Our immune systems are strongly supported by a healthy diet. The immune system prevents infections and diseases posed by harmful foreign bacteria, viruses, and toxins. These are called antigens, and we are all exposed to them every day. They come from the air we breathe, items we touch, and the food and water we consume.

The immune system's first line of defense against antigens is our skin. In addition, key organs and organ systems have mucus membrane linings. Both our skin and mucus linings are physical barriers that help prevent antigens from entering our bodies.

If an antigen gets past these barriers, the immune system defends against it using various types of white blood cells and antibodies. These attack and eliminate the antigens. These defenses are supported by our gut microbiota, lymph cells, spleen, and bone marrow.

The white blood cells and antibodies are transported through our circulatory systems via blood to infected areas. Blood vessels in these areas expand from the additional blood. This is called **inflammation**. Inflammation also helps contain the antigen, keeping it from spreading to other parts of the body. It typically dissipates once the antigen is destroyed.

Immunity health problems include chronic inflammation, arthritis, asthma, allergies, and immune deficiencies. Their primary causes are genetics, aging, lifestyle, medication use, illness, and poor diet.

These immunity health issues are beyond the scope of this book, but I do want to highlight **chronic inflammation.** This health condition has been growing in tandem with metabolic syndrome globally.

Chronic inflammation occurs when the body continues its inflammation response even after there is no infection or disease. It can last for months or even years. Chronic inflammation increases the risk for several chronic conditions, including cancer, cardiovascular disease, stroke, type 2 diabetes, arthritis, and liver disease.

The risk of chronic inflammation increases as we age. In addition to poor diet, the condition is believed to result from lifestyle issues such as high stress levels, poor sleep, smoking, excessive alcohol consumption, and not exercising.

Diet-related health issues such as obesity, an unhealthy microbiota, and oxidative stress are all highly associated with chronic inflammation. In addition, regular consumption of highly processed foods with high levels of sodium, added sugar, and saturated fats is believed to increase the risk of this condition.

A key strategy for a healthy immune system is a diverse, nutrient-dense diet. Certain macronutrients, micronutrients, phytonutrients, antioxidants, and fiber are all particularly essential for our immune system to function properly.

Specifically, consuming healthy levels of protein helps with microbiota gut lining health and immune cell growth and production. Polyunsaturated fat omega-3s and omega-6s are important for maintaining proper levels of inflammation. Lastly, vitamins A, several Bs, C, D and E, and the minerals zinc, selenium, and iron are all important for a healthy immune system.

In the next two sections, I will describe these nutrients in detail and identify those that are particularly helpful to our immune systems.

Metabolic Syndrome and Obesity

This section would not be complete without describing metabolic syndrome. A person has this syndrome when they have three of five adverse health conditions. These conditions are excess body weight, high triglyceride levels, low HDL levels, high blood sugar, and high blood pressure. The medical community has separately defined metabolic syndrome because these health conditions tend to occur concurrently.

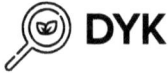

⊘ DYK

It is estimated that one-third of all Americans now have metabolic syndrome, and this number is growing. [34]

Diet and exercise are the two key strategies recommended by most health experts to prevent or reduce the effects of metabolic syndrome.

Obesity is a specific chronic condition highly correlated with metabolic syndrome. According to the CDC, from the early 1960s to 2017, the American adult obesity rate more than tripled, from 13% to 42%. For children and adolescents, the rate quadrupled, from 5% to 20%. Given the current U.S. population, this would translate to over 100 million adults and 15 million children/adolescents.[35]

Obesity is highly associated with many other serious health risks, including cardiovascular disease, stroke, diabetes, inflammation, numerous types of cancer, kidney disease, cognitive brain dysfunction, depression, birth complications, infertility, respiratory diseases, and shorter lifespan.

🔍 DYK

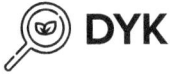

Studies estimate that the obese are 10x more likely to have type 2 diabetes than the non-obese. [36]

There are several studies linking obesity and increased consumption of highly processed foods. As mentioned above, these foods often add high amounts of unhealthy ingredients and preservatives. The good news: Studies show that even modest weight loss can have a significantly positive impact on reducing some of these health risks.

One of the key strategies for weight loss is to transition from highly processed foods to a diet of fresh meats and whole plant foods. These foods include lean proteins, complex carbohydrates, healthy unsaturated fats, vitamins, and important minerals. All these nutrients support weight management.

Additional sources used for immune system, metabolic syndrome and obesity descriptions: [37] [38] [39] [40] [41] [42] [43] [44] [45]

SECTION I KEY TAKEAWAYS

- Humans evolved to consume diets comprised of a variety of wild fresh meats and whole plant foods. These foods contain the essential macronutrients and micronutrients needed for good health.

- To function properly, our bodies require a consistent intake of these nutrients at recommended daily levels. Our digestive systems, gut microbiota, metabolisms, immune systems, brain functions, and energy levels all rely heavily on these nutrients.

- Regularly consuming highly processed foods, which contain unnaturally high levels of sugar, sodium, saturated fats, and calories, can result in severe health issues, including several chronic conditions.

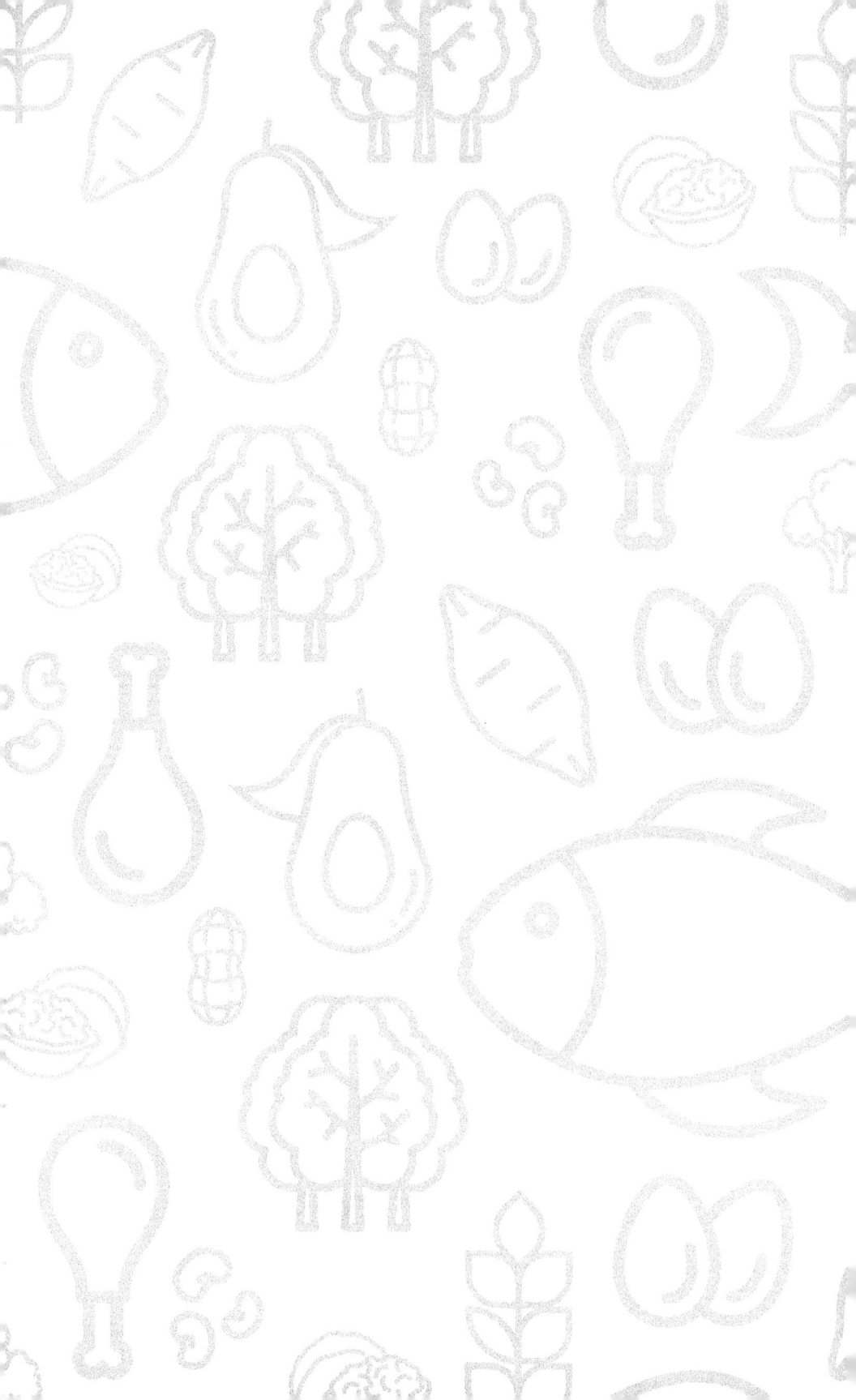

SECTION II

Macronutrients

With Section I's background, let's now go into more detail on key individual nutrients. As a reminder, dietary nutrition is broken down into three primary categories: macronutrients, micronutrients, and a new area called phytonutrients. This section focuses on macronutrients.

The three macronutrients are proteins, carbohydrates, and fats. We need to consume these in relatively large amounts compared to micronutrients. They are considered essential because our bodies do not produce them or do not produce them in sufficient quantities for good health. We must get them from our diet.

I recommend a diet strategy that focuses on nutrient-dense foods to ensure you get recommended amounts of macronutrients and micronutrients. If you regularly consume these foods, there is no need to count or stress about getting your daily nutrients. A strategy counting nutrients is just too complicated and too much effort for most of us. I believe few people would be able to sustain such a diet strategy throughout their lifetimes.

The chapters in this section provide a general description of each of the three macronutrients, their health purpose, related health risks, and recommended daily amounts. Unfortunately, the U.S. government's daily recommendations on macronutrient levels can be confusing or, in some cases, missing completely. In addition to protein, fats, and carbohydrates, there are numerous macronutrient subcategories. These are all also described in this section.

To simplify things, I have tried throughout this section to eliminate scientific jargon and recommend simple approaches to attain healthy levels of daily macronutrients. Even with this simplification, some of the explanations may be difficult to digest (pun intended). Please don't worry about trying to translate all these daily recommendations into your diet. The later sections on foods and meals will help with this. For now, just try to get a basic understanding of macronutrients and their importance for our health.

Before starting, below is some background information on daily nutrient recommendations that will help you better understand this section and the next.

Nutrient recommendations are made in the U.S. by the Food and Nutrition Board (FNB). It recommends specific daily amounts for individual macronutrients and micronutrients. To determine these recommendations, it evaluates the science on each nutrient's health impact. If credible science shows that a nutrient is essential for good health and has a critical role in preventing disease or supporting a key body function, a daily recommendation is made.

When the FNB establishes a daily nutrient intake recommendation (called a Dietary Reference Intake or DRI), there are three different levels that can be given. The level depends on the degree to which the science demonstrates the nutrient's health impact. These are described as:

- **Recommended Dietary Allowance (RDA):** Daily nutrient intake level sufficient to meet the requirements of 97–98% of healthy individuals.
- **Adequate Intake (AI):** When available evidence is not sufficient to determine an RDA, then an AI is set for a nutrient.
- **Estimated Average Requirement (EAR):** Daily nutrient intake level expected to meet the requirement of 50% of healthy individuals.

These are commonly used acronyms in many nutrition publications. You don't have to memorize these DRIs, but please know that regardless of level assigned, all of these are the FNB's best advice on the daily nutrient amounts needed for good health.

As you will see, some important nutrients do not have a daily recommendation because the science is not at the level to make one.

You may also see the term **Tolerable Upper Intake Level (UL)** used in this chapter and on some nutrient supplement labels. This is the FNB's recommended highest daily intake level of a nutrient before adverse health risks can result. This limit is used primarily for supplements and medications, as it is very rare to have negative health impacts from foods with high nutrient levels.

Why are all these DRI recommendations important? Because they create daily nutrient targets for a healthy diet. To keep things simple, I use the acronym DRI for any daily recommendation I describe.

Macronutrient and micronutrient measurements can sometimes be confusing due to their varying terminology. It's important to understand these measurements so the dietary strategies recommended later make sense.

Credible nutritional information sources, like the FNB, use the metric system to measure macronutrients, micronutrients, and phytonutrients. The basic measure starts with grams.

One ounce equals approximately 28 grams. So, a gram is a small amount! Almost all macronutrients in this section, and their related nutrients, are measured in grams. [46] [47]

With this background, let's now dive into the individual macronutrients.

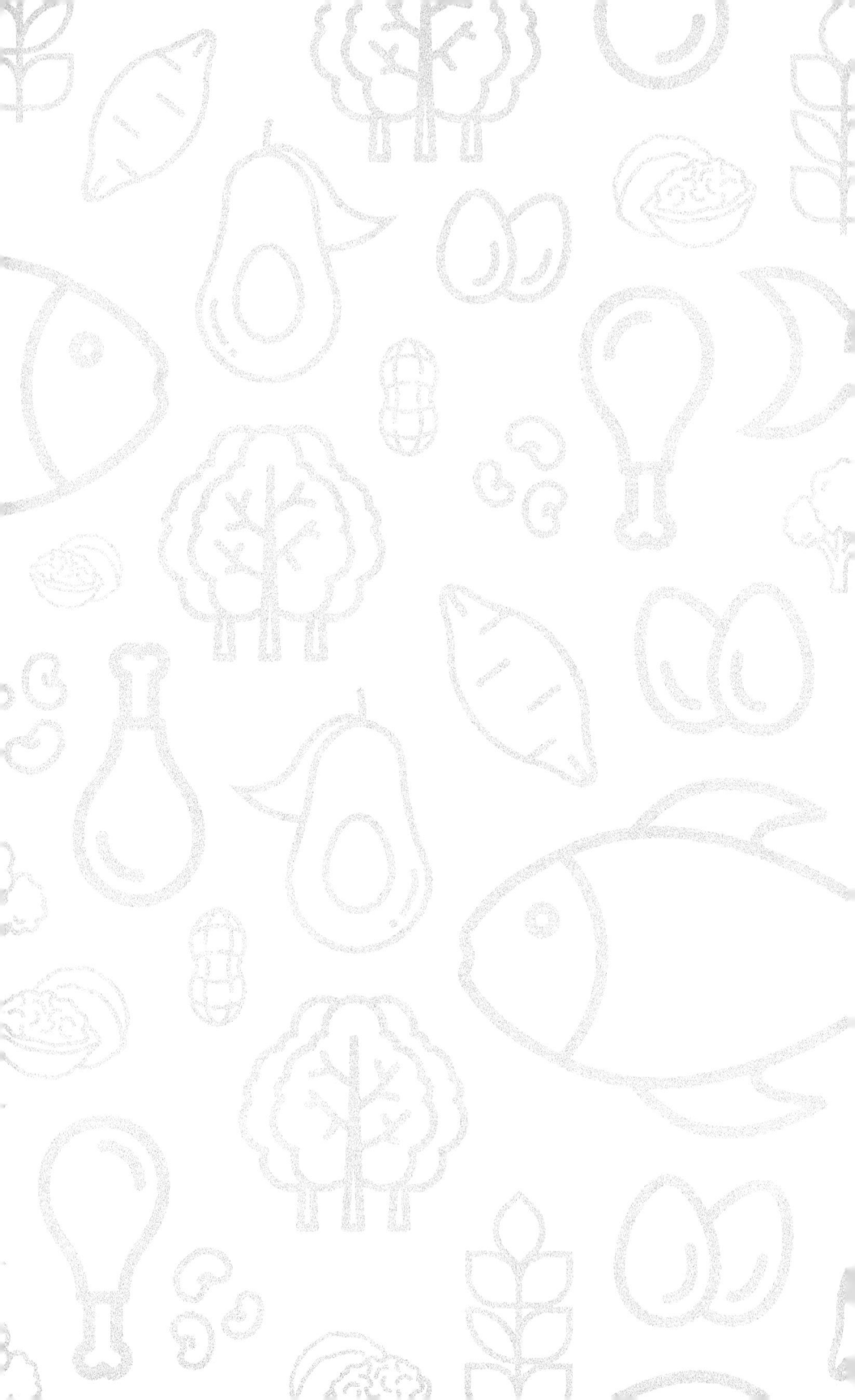

CHAPTER 5

Proteins

Dietary protein has enjoyed a great deal of popularity over the last few decades. While this popularity is primarily due to its support of weight loss and muscle gain, protein has many other important health functions.

Protein has a key role in building, maintaining, and repairing important body structures. In addition to muscles, protein supports our bones, brains, organs, hair, skin, and all cell membranes.

Other types of proteins, like enzymes, antibodies, and hormones, support important metabolic reactions. These include maintaining the body's pH balance, strengthening its immune system, and transporting and storing nutrients.

Protein Health Risks

Health issues related to proteins can come from consuming either too little protein or from frequently consuming protein foods with high levels of saturated fats. The health risks from high saturated fats are covered in the fats and fatty acids chapter below.

In terms of protein inadequacy, most Americans consume up to current recommended levels, but some population groups do not. Older Americans are one such demographic group. Surveys show that a significant percentage of adults over age 50 consume less than the daily recommendation. Also, our digestive systems tend to be less effective in absorbing proteins and other nutrients as we age.

Low protein intake and absorption can lead to significant reductions in bone density and muscle loss for the elderly. These low levels increase the risks of osteoporosis and sarcopenia.[48] Low protein levels are also believed to adversely affect normal brain function.[49]

Osteoporosis is characterized by significant bone loss, reduced bone strength, and an increased risk of bone fractures. A chronic disease, osteoporosis affects over 10 million people in the U.S. over 50. Further, approximately 50 million more Americans have low bone mass, which increases their risk for osteoporosis. The condition of low bone mass is called **osteopenia**.[50]

Sarcopenia is characterized by loss of muscle mass, strength, and function. Approximately 18% of Americans over 60 have below-normal muscle strength. This number exceeds 50% by age 80. Sarcopenia symptoms include muscle weakness, fatigue, balance problems, and trouble walking and standing. It also increases the risk of falls resulting in bone fractures.[51]

Low protein levels can also affect **brain function**. Protein is an important nutrient for the brain to build and maintain its neurotransmitters. Studies of the elderly show that low protein intake is associated with **mild cognitive impairment** and potentially **dementia**.

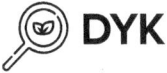

DYK

Excluding water, protein comprises 80% of muscle mass, over 30% of bone mass, and 35% of brain mass.[52]

Consuming the daily recommended amount of protein significantly reduces the risk of these medical conditions. Several studies also recommend the elderly consume even higher levels of protein than the current U.S. recommendations, in order to prevent or delay the onset of brain health issues.

Consuming unhealthy, high amounts of protein is rare in the U.S. There is no FNB daily UL for protein. Consuming too much protein is difficult, as it's very filling, especially if you are eating a balanced diet full of plant and animal foods. If you do consume excessive amounts of protein, studies show you are at higher risk of kidney stones and issues with your digestive system.

🏅 Pro Move

Does it matter the time of day you consume protein? Yes! Americans get most of their protein at dinner. Yet studies show our bodies can only absorb approximately 20–40 grams of protein per meal. Research indicates that evenly consuming protein throughout all meals is the best way for the body to fully absorb it and reach healthy daily levels.

Daily Protein Intake Recommendations

Unfortunately, the U.S. daily protein recommendations are confusing. The FNB makes two recommendations for daily protein. A DRI of .36 grams of protein per pound of body weight, and daily protein levels at 10–35% of calories.

Two observations on the FNB gram recommendation. First, it is based on science from over 80 years ago. Second, for most people it translates to protein levels below the FNB's own percentage range of calories. I have not found a reasonable explanation for this disconnect, and the error has been identified by several credible nutritional sources.

Putting this discrepancy aside, my research suggests that this protein gram-based DRI is too low. Healthy, active adults need higher levels. I recommend you consume **.5–.9 grams of daily protein per pound of body weight.** The range is based on your activity level.

This recommendation is based on a study by The American College of Sports Medicine and the Academy of Nutrition and Dietitians of Canada. It recommends that active people consume up to .9 grams of protein per pound of body weight each day. There are several other credible studies recommending protein ranges similar to this one or, in some cases, even higher.[53]

If you are very active, go with the higher end of this range. If sedentary, then the lower end should meet your daily protein needs. Also, if you are elderly, it's important that you stay within this range consistently. As noted above, numerous studies show the elderly do not consume adequate levels of protein.

Determining Your Protein Grams

What does this daily protein recommendation equal in terms of grams for the average American? Well, an adult female at average height, activity level, and weight should consume between 63–112 grams of daily protein, or an average of approximately 90 grams.

An adult male at average height, activity level, and weight would need 75–135 grams of protein. This would average 105 grams of daily protein. These averages calculate to over 15% of daily calories, which is well within the FNB's protein range recommendation of 10–35% of daily calories.

For the purposes of establishing a daily protein benchmark for this book, I used 100 grams. This basically averages the midpoint of the female and male target ranges above. I use this benchmark to evaluate the protein levels of all foods and meals described in the book.

Note that there are several online tools to calculate your individual daily calorie and nutrient needs; I describe one at the beginning of Section V. This will provide more specific recommendations for your daily caloric and nutrition needs, but as you will see I do not believe it is necessary to use such tools. If you are eating a diet consistent with my food and meal recommendations in Sections IV and V, you will get the calories and nutrition at levels your body needs for good health (including protein).

My Daily Protein Approach

Based on my research for this book, I upgraded my diet with higher levels of daily protein. I'm an active person that regularly lifts weights, walks, and participates in sports. At age 62, I need to make sure I'm getting enough protein to support my active lifestyle. I do not count my daily protein grams (or calories). For me, consuming the right foods, as described later in the book, is the best strategy for getting adequate protein.

I rely on the foods in my diet to help me consume approximately 30–40 grams of protein per meal. My goal is to reach a minimum of 100 grams of protein daily. This works out to be over .6 grams of protein per pound of my body weight, or 16% of my theoretical daily calorie target. The foods I focus on for healthy levels of protein are fatty fish, chicken, eggs, legumes, and whole-wheat bread.

Note that if you have kidney health issues, you should consult a physician before changing your protein intake.

Protein Facts Break

→ *There are over 10,000 different proteins in our bodies and they make up approximately 20% of our bodies' weight.*

→ *Unlike carbohydrates and fats, the body doesn't store much protein. You need to consume adequate levels every day.*

→ *The body uses proteins as an energy source as a last resort after glucose (carbohydrates) and triglycerides (fats) are exhausted.*

→ *Crickets are one of the highest sources of protein in the animal kingdom. Bon appetit!*

Additional sources used for protein description: [54] [55] [56] [57] [58] [59] [60] [61] [62] [63] [64]

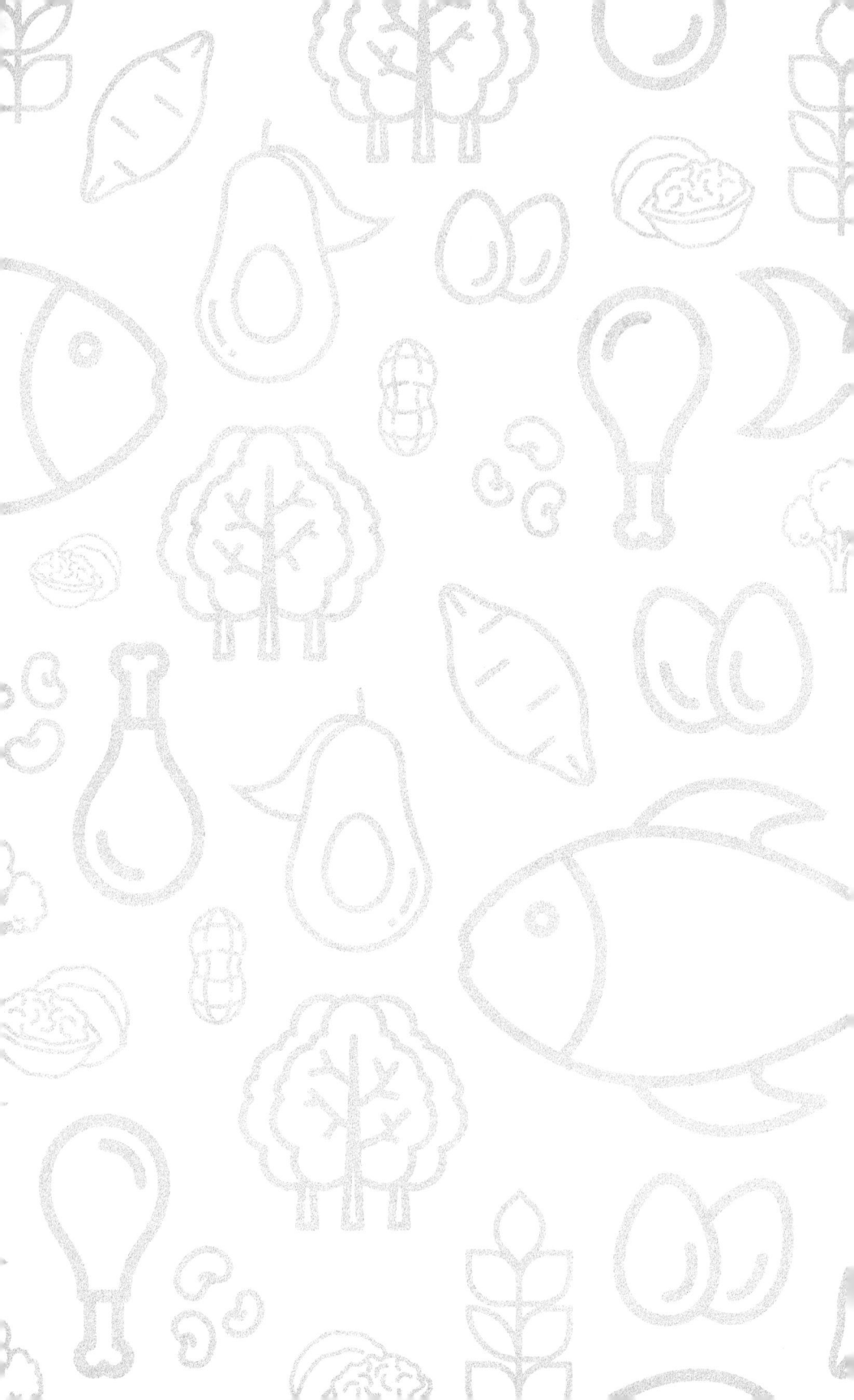

CHAPTER 6

Fats

Historically, fats have an undeserved bad reputation. For many years, fats were shunned because they were thought to make us fat. In truth, there are several different types of dietary fats, with mostly positive and some negative impacts on our health.

As described in Section I, dietary fats include saturated, polyunsaturated, and monounsaturated fats. All dietary fats are turned into fatty acids during digestion and, eventually, into triglycerides. These are transferred into the bloodstream as a lipoprotein. Our cells use these triglycerides for energy.

Cholesterol is another type of blood lipid but is mostly produced by our livers, with only small amounts coming from our foods. Its purpose is to maintain cell membranes and produce essential hormones. There are two forms of blood cholesterol, LDL (the "bad" kind) and HDL (the "good" kind).

Types of Dietary Fat and Potential Health Risks

There are several different dietary fats. You should know that all dietary fats are part of a natural, healthy diet except for trans fats.

Saturated fats are found in many animal foods, certain oils, and even in low amounts in most plant foods. The best health strategy for saturated fat is to limit your intake to recommended levels.

Health issues related to saturated fats come from consuming too many foods high in these fats. Highly processed foods often contain unnaturally high levels of saturated fats. High levels are also contained in several animal foods, particularly red meat. Studies show diets high in some of these foods raise both bloodstream triglycerides and LDL cholesterol to unhealthy levels.

High LDL levels have been shown to cause plaque buildup in blood vessel walls. This buildup narrows these vessels and makes them more rigid. This condition, called **atherosclerosis**, can lead to high blood pressure and is associated with several cardiovascular diseases.

High blood pressure (also called hypertension) can also result from consuming high levels of sodium. **Hypertension** raises the risk of several cardiovascular health problems. Nearly half the U.S. adult population, or approximately 120 million people, have hypertension.[65]

Hypertension is also associated with health issues like type 2 diabetes, fatty liver disease, kidney disease, vision problems, pancreatitis, inflammation, and metabolic syndrome. As we age, our blood pressure tends to increase, so monitoring saturated fat and sodium intake levels becomes even more important.

Cardiovascular disease, which includes heart attack and stroke, is strongly associated with high levels of triglycerides and LDL cholesterol in the bloodstream. Cardiovascular disease alone kills approximately 900,000 Americans annually.[66]

Some recent studies have questioned previous findings that high saturated fat intake causes heart disease. However, these newer studies do not seem to question whether such diets cause high LDL levels, atherosclerosis, and high blood pressure. It's a rather confusing scientific argument, but one that means more credible studies are needed for this important issue.

Unfortunately, several studies show that over two-thirds of Americans consume more than the recommended daily saturated fat level. A key health goal for our diets is to make sure we consume saturated fats at or below these levels. Just as important, we need to consistently consume recommended levels of unsaturated fats.[67]

While overconsumption of saturated fats is associated with cardiovascular disease, consuming unsaturated fats within recommended levels helps to reduce the risk.[68] [69] [70] [71] [72] [73] [74]

Unsaturated fats are divided into polyunsaturated and monounsaturated fats. **Polyunsaturated fats** (**PUFAs**) are commonly referred to as omega-3 and omega-6 fatty acids. Our bodies don't make these nutrients, so we must get them from our diet. Although there are several types of **omega-3s**, the three

most well-known are alpha-linolenic acid (ALA), eicosatetrae-
noic acid (EPA), and docosahexaenoic acid (DHA).

Omega-3 ALA, or linolenic acid, comes from plant foods
such as walnuts, chia seeds, kale, and soybeans. Credible studies
associate omega-3 ALA consumption with positive impacts on
cardiovascular health, inflammation, and depression.

ALA also converts into omega-3 EPA and DHA in our
bodies. It is believed that less than 10% of ALA is converted, so
while omega-3 ALA is healthy, it does not seem to have the same
direct health benefits of omega-3 EPA and DHA.

Omega-3 EPA and DHA primarily come from consuming
fatty fish such as salmon and some shellfish. These fatty acids
are found in high concentrations in our brains and eyes and are
believed to be important for the bodies' cell membrane structures.

Studies show an association between these omega-3s and
lower triglyceride levels, lower risk of cardiovascular disease,
healthy brain function, better blood flow in the brain, lower
inflammation, and better eye health. These fatty acids may also
be helpful with the treatment of depression and in reducing the
symptoms of dementia.

DYK

*Approximately 20% of brain weight is comprised of omega-3s,
primarily omega-3 DHA.*[75]

A recent study has also found an association between high omega-3 intake and the slowing of aging. More research is needed on this important nutrient.

Omega-6 fatty acids can be found at high levels in chicken thighs and legs, sardines, eggs, most tree nuts, peanuts/peanut butter, soybeans/soy products, avocados, 100% whole-wheat bread, quinoa, olive oil, pumpkin and chia seeds, and certain cooking oils. The most common omega-6 in our foods is called linoleic acid.

Studies show that omega-6 fatty acids support reduced LDL and triglyceride levels and promote healthy cell structures and cell processes.

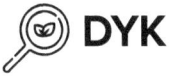

DYK

A few studies have raised health concerns about omega-6 fatty acids causing inflammation, but this opinion is not supported by many credible medical organizations. For example, the American Heart Association has stated that omega-6 fatty acids are safe and good for cardiovascular health. [76]

Studies show that, on average, U.S. adults do not consume enough polyunsaturated fats. As you can see from all their health benefits, we need to make sure we get more unprocessed foods with these fats into our diets.

Monounsaturated fats (MUFAs) are another healthy unsaturated fat. Examples of foods high in monounsaturated fats include avocados, peanuts, most tree nuts, olive oil, olives, and most animal foods. One word of caution: animal foods high in monounsaturated fat also tend to be even higher in saturated fat. Be careful with your source of monounsaturated fats.

The most common monounsaturated fat in our foods is oleic acid. Regular consumption of this fat is associated with many health benefits, including increased HDL levels. HDL is considered a healthy lipid and shown to lower LDL levels.

Some studies state that plant-based sources of mono-unsaturated fats resulted in the greatest health benefits. As with other unsaturated fats, more research is needed on this important nutrient.

Trans fats are the last type of dietary unsaturated fat. These fats are commonly found in highly processed foods such as cakes, cookies, microwave popcorn, frozen pizza, refrigerated biscuits and rolls, fried foods like French fries and doughnuts, non-dairy coffee creamer, shortening, and margarine.

Trans fats are universally accepted as unhealthy, as they are shown in studies to raise LDL levels and lower HDL levels. Trans fats increase the risk of cardiovascular disease and type 2 diabetes. The U.S. Food and Drug Administration (FDA) has taken steps to reduce trans fats from being added to foods.

Check the nutrition facts labels of your foods to see if they contain trans fats or partially hydrogenated oils. If so, please try to avoid these foods.

Daily Fats Intake Recommendations

It's important to consume a diet high in unsaturated fats and only at or below recommended levels of saturated fats. If you do this, you're getting critical dietary macronutrients that help you maintain long-term health. Note that the FNB has not made recommendations for all of the fats described below.

Total daily fats target: The FNB recommends **total daily fats at 20–35% of daily calories**. This is supported by almost all credible health information sources. Based on the average American's profile, as described in the protein chapter, the total daily fats intake should be approximately 70 grams for females and 85 grams for males.

Saturated fat: The FNB recommends consuming saturated fats at less than 10% of daily calories. The American Heart Association (AHA) recommends a lower limit of 6% of daily calories.[77]

I used a **saturated fat target of under 10% of daily calories** as the benchmark for my food and meal analyses in Sections IV and V. For the average American, this translates to a daily saturated fat level less than 25 grams for females and less than 30 grams for males.

Based on the FNB's 10% daily calorie limit, the remainder of our fats should come from unsaturated fats. On average, this would mean that we should consume nearly twice as much unsaturated fat as saturated fat. This translates to approximately 45–55 grams of unsaturated fats daily.

I was unable to find a credible health organization that specifically supports this 2:1 unsaturated to saturated fat ratio. This is likely because of the lack of studies on this nutrition issue.

Nonetheless, most credible health sources state that we should regularly consume more unsaturated fat than saturated fat. For the remainder of the book, I use the 2:1 unsaturated to saturated ratio as a benchmark for whether a food or meal has a healthy fat profile.

Unsaturated fats: The FNB recommends daily levels for omega-3 ALA and omega-6 but has no recommendations for omega-3 EPA and DHA or monounsaturated fats.

Omega-3 ALA and Omega-6 fatty acids: I support the FNB's recommended **daily omega-3-ALA intake of 1.1–1.6 grams** and **omega-6 at 12–17 grams**. These ranges are based on an adults' gender. I use these as the benchmark for my food and meal analyses.[78] [79]

Omega-3 EPA and DHA fatty acids: Given the potential health benefits of these omega-3s, it is a real nutritional miss by the FNB not to make a recommendation. Fortunately, several credible health and nutrition organizations recommend a total for these two fatty acids of between 250–500 milligrams daily.

The AHA goes further and recommends 2–3 grams of these fats per day. The FDA stated that it's safe to consume up to 5 grams of these omega-3's daily (via both food and supplements).[80] [81]

With this background, I recommend **2–3 grams of daily omega-3 EPA and DHA** as a nutritional target. While more research is needed, these fats have shown in studies to be incredibly important to brain health and warrant using a higher, but safe, level for a daily intake target.

🏅 Pro Move

If you're not a fish or seafood fan, try a fish oil supplement with omega-3 EPA/DHA. Make sure to read the nutrition facts label to ensure the supplement provides healthy amounts of daily EPA and DHA.

Monosaturated fats: I could find no credible guidance for daily monounsaturated fat intake, although many medical associations, nutrition experts, and studies espouse the health benefits of these fats.

Using the recommendations for the other unsaturated fats and the 2:1 fat profile ratio described above, a range of 30–35 grams or approximately 12% of daily calories would be reasonable. As a point of reference, if you consumed one-half of a medium-sized avocado, a handful of walnuts, 2 tablespoons of flax seeds, and 2 tablespoons of olive oil daily, you would get approximately 30–35 grams of monounsaturated fats. Most health experts support the daily consumption of these foods and recommend them as part of a healthy diet.

I recommend **monounsaturated fat at approximately 12% of daily calories or 30–35 grams** and use this level as a benchmark for a healthy diet.

Trans fats: The FNB recommends avoiding foods with trans fats as much as possible, unless you have food access issues. The AHA recommends intake of less than 1% of daily calories, which for most of us would be under 2 grams. I agree with this target of **trans fats at less than 1% of daily calories**.

My Daily Fats Approach

While added sugar (covered in the next chapter) is likely the top dietary health risk for Americans, I have always thought of saturated fat as my personal biggest health risk. I've had several family members experience early death or have severe health issues related to heart attacks and stroke.

Growing up, my southern U.S. family consumed what was then considered a healthy diet, but as I think back, many of the foods we consumed were very high in saturated fat. Also, we had virtually no understanding of unsaturated fats.

Foods high in unsaturated fats like avocados, olives, seeds, salmon, and whole-wheat grains were just not part of our menu options. Our diet was not entirely without unsaturated fats, as we did regularly consume chicken, tree nuts, and eggs.

Because of my family's health issues, for most of my adult life I shied away from what I thought were foods high in saturated fat foods. This probably helped keep my cholesterol at healthy levels. However, I now know I likely wasn't getting sufficient levels of omega-3s and monounsaturated fats.

I have changed this by getting recommended levels of these important unsaturated fats through regularly consuming more fatty fish and avocados, mostly using olive oil for cooking, and taking a daily omega-3 EPA/DHA supplement. Fortunately, all my cardiovascular health measures have been very good to date.

The foods and meals I recommend in the later sections will help you limit your saturated fat intake to safe levels and achieve recommended levels of unsaturated fats. All the meals I describe in Section V have very healthy unsaturated to saturated fat ratios. Most are well over the 2:1 ratio described above.

Additional sources used for fats description: [82] [83] [84] [85] [86] [87] [88] [89] [90] [91] [92] [93] [94] [95] [96]

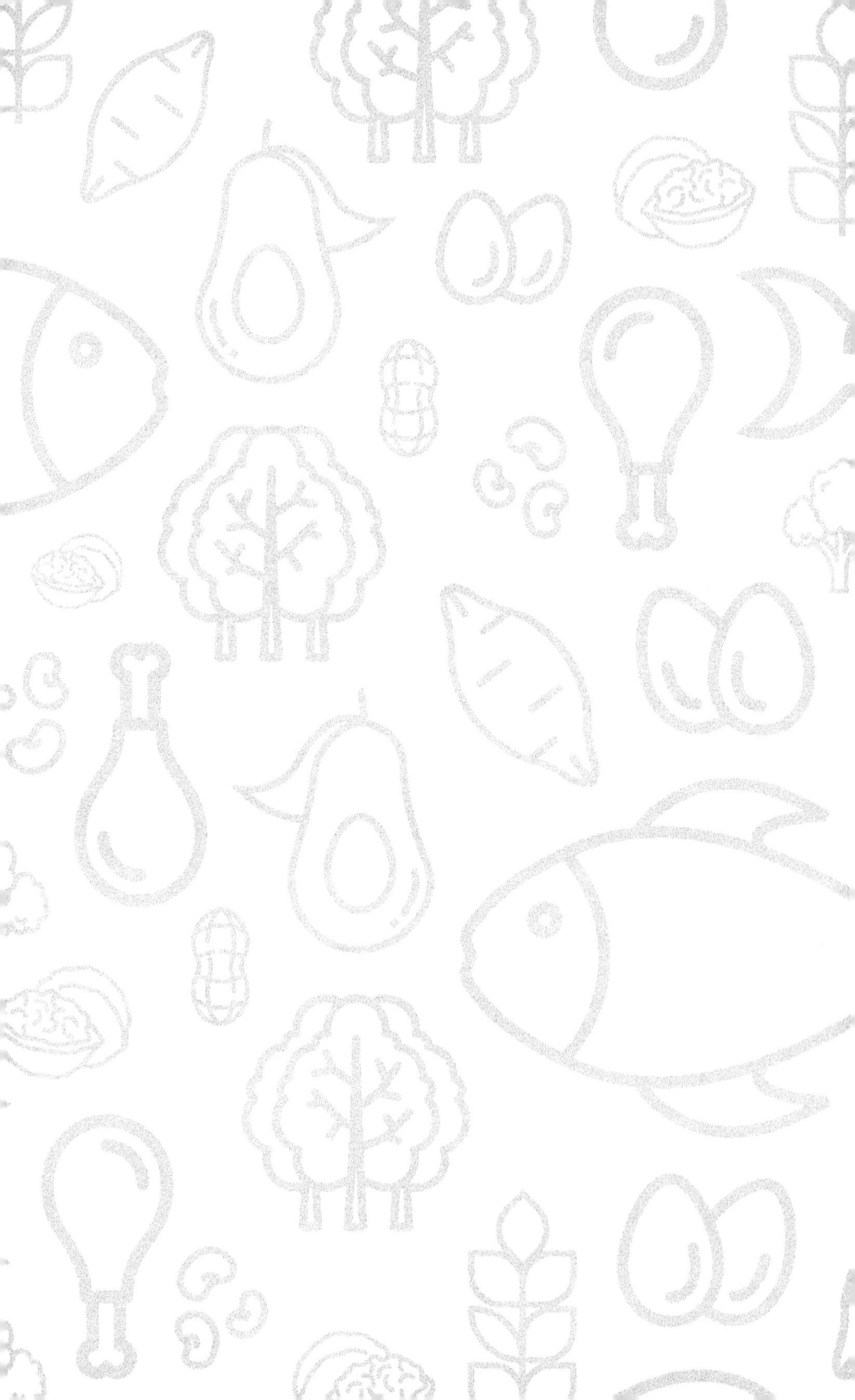

CHAPTER 7

Carbohydrates

Carbohydrates ("carbs") are another misunderstood macronutrient. They have an undeserved reputation for causing weight gain and blood sugar problems. It is true that certain carb foods can cause these health issues. However, by selecting healthy, whole plant foods for our carbohydrates, we get important nutrients and a great source of energy and reduce our chances of obesity and diabetes.

Carbs are our body's primary source of daily energy. Note that most animal foods have no carbohydrates or very low amounts.

Types of Carbohydrates and Potential Health Risks

Complex carbohydrates contain sugars, fiber, and sometimes starch. Complex carbohydrates are naturally contained in vegetables, fruits, legumes, nuts, whole grains, and seeds. Studies show that we do not consume enough of these healthy carb foods.

During digestion, these foods' sugars and starches are broken down into single sugar molecules, primarily **glucose**.

This occurs in the small intestine, and the glucose is transferred into the bloodstream.

This glucose is in a form that can be used by our cells for energy. When glucose is released into the bloodstream, insulin is also released by the pancreas, and this allows the glucose to enter our cells for energy use.

Starch in complex carbs is comprised of long chains of sugar molecules. This chain structure causes digestion to take longer. While foods with starch can have high amounts of sugar, the slower digestion helps reduce the risk of spikes in blood sugar and insulin levels.

Fiber has a similar digestive effect as starch and is a very important nutrient for our overall health. Fiber consists of the indigestible cellulose in plant cell walls and other plant materials. This indigestible material also slows the digestion of complex carbohydrate foods.

Fiber's slow digestion not only supports healthy blood sugar levels, but also a healthy gut microbiota. An added health benefit is that it helps us stay full longer which reduces overeating.

There are two types of fiber, soluble and insoluble.

Soluble fiber turns into a gel-like substance during digestion and has been shown to not only slow the absorption of glucose but also lower the absorption of dietary fats and cholesterol. In addition, soluble fiber is a prebiotic (food source) for our gut microbiota bacteria.

Insoluble fiber is not digestible. It passes through the digestive tract into the large intestine. While not a prebiotic, this type of fiber supports a healthy digestive tract.

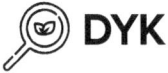

🔍 DYK

On average Americans consume only half the recommended amount of daily fiber. Further, national surveys indicate approximately 95% of Americans do not meet this recommended level. The overconsumption of highly processed foods is one reason for Americans' low fiber intake.[97]

Simple carbohydrate foods are often highly processed and have high amounts of sugar added. They contain little or no fiber and starch. Examples of these foods include baked sweets, candy, pizza, refined grain breads, many breakfast cereals and soft drinks and energy drinks.

Added sugar deserves to be highlighted here. It is a significant health risk to Americans and people worldwide. Added sugar is not a natural ingredient in foods and provides little nutritional value. It is often referred to as empty calories.

Health issues related to carbohydrates primarily come from regularly consuming highly processed simple carb foods. With little to no fiber or starch, the added sugars in these foods are digested quickly, resulting in glucose's swift release into the bloodstream. This can cause a rapid rise in blood sugar levels.

Frequent blood sugar spikes lead to frequent insulin releases. Over time, this can make our cells resistant to insulin. This resistance interferes with the cells' ability to absorb and metabolize the glucose for energy.

This condition, called **insulin resistance**, can cause blood glucose to rise to unhealthy levels. Consistently high blood sugar is called **hyperglycemia**. Over time, persistent hyperglycemia can lead to prediabetes and, eventually, type 2 diabetes.

Conversely, complex carbohydrate foods do not increase the risk of these health issues and are important for good health and energy. As described above, the fiber and starch slow digestion, resulting in fewer glucose spikes; they also support a healthy gut microbiota and digestive system.

Type 2 diabetes affects approximately 35 million U.S. adults, and over 84 million adults are prediabetic. This means their blood sugar is elevated but not quite high enough to be considered diabetic.[98] [99]

Diabetes and prediabetes rates are increasing. Among U.S. children and adolescents, type 2 diabetes has nearly doubled in the last 15 years, reaching rates of 18%. There is no cure for type 2 diabetes.[100]

Many credible studies show that added sugar is a major cause of type 2 diabetes. Added sugar also increases the risks of obesity, inflammation, cardiovascular disease, and depression, and negatively affects brain health. It is further associated with osteoporosis, low energy levels, poor dental health, acne, skin aging, cellular aging, fatty liver, and some cancers.

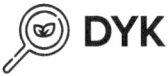

⊚ DYK

Also note that excess sugar can cause our livers to become overloaded with glucose which, at high levels, is converted into triglycerides. This is thought to be a primary cause of obesity.

The bottom line is that we all need to limit simple carbohydrate foods and added sugar in our diets. Please read the nutrition facts labels to understand how much added sugar is in your food. Try to select foods with no or very low amounts of added sugar.

Daily Carbohydrate Intake Recommendations

Total carbohydrates target: The FNB recommends **45–65% carbohydrate range for daily calories**, a range that is supported by most credible health organizations. Based on the profile of the average American female and male, as described in the protein chapter, this translates to a daily average of 300 grams for females and 400 grams for males.

I agreed with this daily range until I analyzed the carbohydrate levels in the healthy foods described in Section IV. What did I find? At typical serving sizes, it is virtually impossible to reach this daily carb range with healthy, whole plant foods.

Most credible health experts recommend that diets include a variety of natural, whole, unprocessed plant foods to get your daily complex carbohydrates. These experts further recommend foods such as quinoa, potatoes, oats, 100% whole-wheat bread, apples, legumes, etc. as the best sources for these carbohydrates. However, at typical serving sizes, these foods individually contain no more than 15% of the daily carb recommendation.

When you use a healthy number of these plant foods in daily meals you simply can't get to the FNB daily carb range. My meal examples in Section V average nearly 15 plant foods daily (significantly more than the typical American diet). When eating a full day of these meals, the carb levels achieved reach only about half of the lower end of the FNB range.

DYK

In a single day, let's say you ate 2 slices of 100% whole-wheat bread, ⅔ cup of quinoa, 1 medium baked potato, ⅔ cups of carrots, 1 cup of mixed berries, and 1 cup of black beans. This is a lot of high-carb foods, but only totals 160 grams of carbs or just over half the lower end of the FNB daily recommended range.[102]

Guess which foods provide a greater chance of reaching the FNB carb levels? If you guessed highly processed foods, you're right! Pretzels, sugary cereals, French fries, doughnuts, soft drinks, flavored yogurts, and bagels are all much higher in carbohydrates than whole plant foods.

Perhaps the FNB assumed that highly processed foods would be part of our regular diets in their analysis. However, I can't recommend anyone regularly consume these foods given how detrimental they are to our health.

So, what's the right amount of carbs to consume? My recommendation is to ignore the FNB range and focus your diet on the whole, unprocessed plant foods listed above to get your carbs. Later in the book, I recommend that you try to get at least 10–15 plant foods in your daily diet. This is a healthy approach to getting your daily carbs.

Fiber: The FNB recommends **14 grams of fiber per 1,000 calories daily**. Most credible health information sources support this recommendation. This translates to 30 grams of daily fiber for females and 36 grams daily for males, and I use this for my benchmark for foods' and meals' nutrient levels.

Added sugar: The FNB recommends less than 10% of daily calories come from added sugar. Surprisingly, this does not calculate to much less than what Americans are currently consuming in added sugar (15 teaspoons a day vs. the current U.S. adult average of 17 teaspoons daily). With the number of Americans suffering from diabetes and obesity, this seems like too high a level to support good health.

The AHA recommends **no more than 6% of daily calories**. Other countries have established even lower added sugar recommendations. I recommend the lower AHA daily target. This translates to approximately 32 grams of added sugar daily for females (8 teaspoons) and 40 grams (10 teaspoons) for males and I use these in the book as the daily benchmark.

Note that in the U.S., there is no daily recommended limit for natural sugars contained in complex carbohydrate foods. There is very little research showing these sugars are a health risk.

The UK does have a recommended limit of 90 grams per day for natural sugar. If you have high blood sugar issues, then you may want to use the UK limit and consult your physician before changing your diet. In the foods and meals analyses in the last two sections of the book, I use the 90-gram benchmark to evaluate the amounts of natural sugar.

My Daily Carbohydrates Approach

My carbohydrate food strategy is a very simple one. I eat a wide variety of whole plant foods (cooked and raw) and try to eliminate foods with added sugar. I think this straightforward strategy provides me with the daily carbohydrates and energy I need for my active lifestyle, gives me the fiber levels for good microbiota and digestive tract health, and reduces my risk of diabetes and weight gain.

As for animal foods, I only eat unprocessed meats that have no sugars or carbs. The one exception is dairy, which does have sugar and carbs. I limit my daily intake of dairy to my recommended levels described later in the book. I only consume plain, unflavored versions of dairy. This keeps the added sugar levels very low.

Try these simple strategies. Your body will thank you!

Additional sources used for carbohydrates description: [103] [104] [105] [106] [107] [108] [109] [110] [111] [112] [113]

SECTION II KEY TAKEAWAYS

- **Protein:** This macronutrient has a key role in building, maintaining, and repairing our muscles, bones, brains, organs, hair, skin, and all cell membranes. Every day, try to achieve the recommended level of .5–.9 grams of protein per pound of body weight. To do so, you will need to consume foods with high protein totals at all three daily meals. For most, 30–40 grams of protein per meal is appropriate.

- **Fats:** Dietary fats are turned into triglycerides, and our bodies use these for energy. Those not used are stored for future energy needs. Unsaturated fats support cardiovascular and brain health, reduce inflammation, help to control blood sugar levels, and lower the risk of depression. Focus on foods that are high in unsaturated fat and moderate in saturated fat. Your daily target should be to consume approximately twice the level of unsaturated fat compared to saturated fat. Saturated fat is a healthy nutrient up to the recommended levels. At higher levels, it is believed to increase the risk for cardiovascular disease and other health issues.

- **Carbohydrates:** Our bodies use carbohydrates converted into glucose as their primary energy source. Try to consume whole, unprocessed plant foods as your main source for carbohydrates. These foods are called complex carbohydrates and contain important fiber and starch. Such carbohydrates help maintain healthy blood sugar levels and support a healthy gut microbiota. Limit or avoid completely highly processed, simple carbohydrate foods high in added sugar in your diet.

- **Read your food's nutrition facts labels:** These labels list your food's protein, fats, carbohydrates, fiber, added sugar levels, and certain other nutrients. These are a key information source for making healthy food decisions.

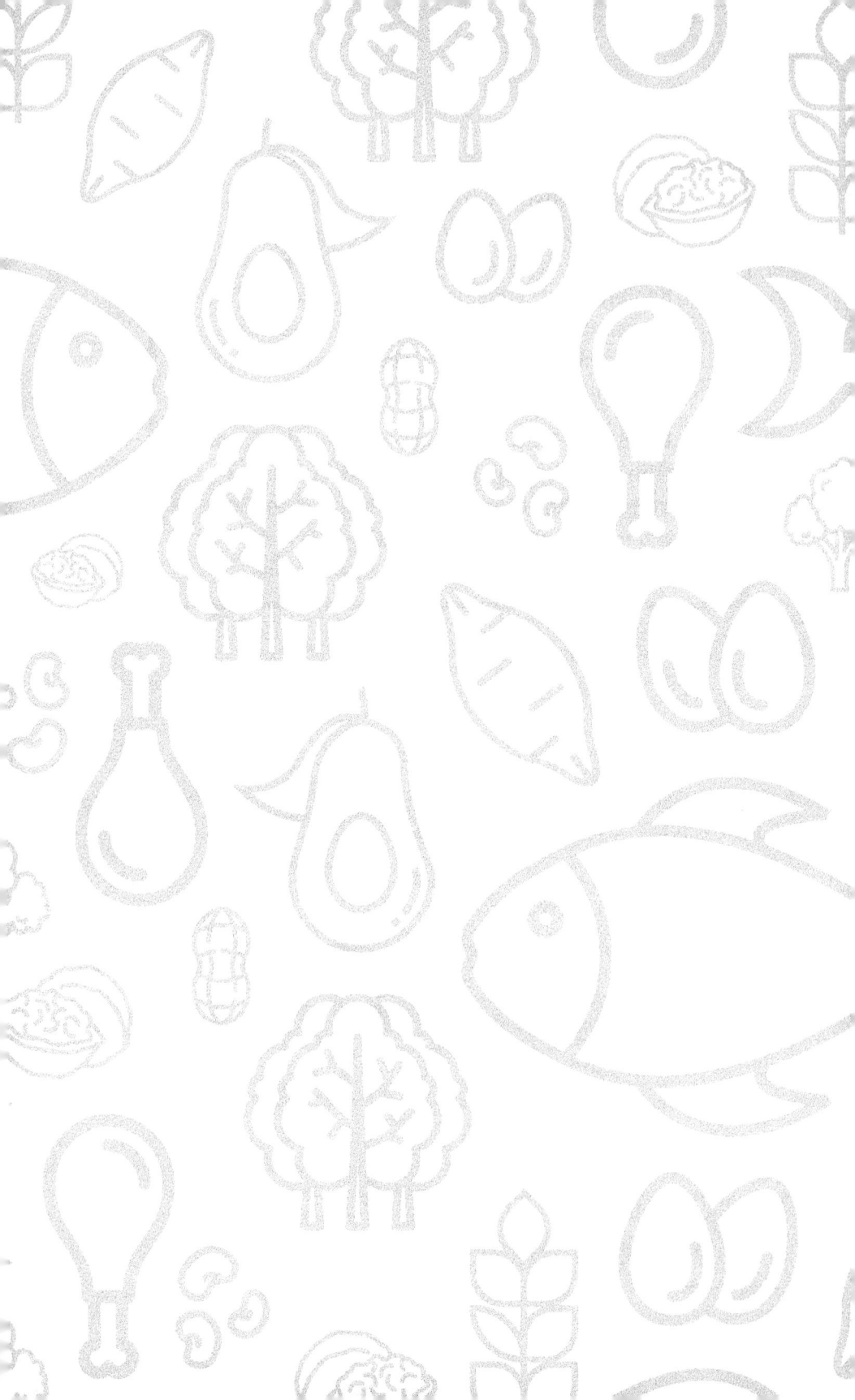

Micronutrients and Phytonutrients

Now that you're an expert on macronutrients, let's turn to micronutrients. These important nutrients should not be forgotten in your daily diet. They offer a broad spectrum of health benefits and support for key body functions, including converting macronutrients into energy; acting as antioxidants; promoting brain and body systems health; and creating new red blood cells, hormones, and enzymes.

Vitamins and minerals are different types of micronutrients. Vitamins are organic substances produced by plants and animals. Minerals are inorganic elements absorbed by plants from earth's rocks, soil, and water.

There are **approximately 30 essential micronutrients** that support our bodies every day. These are considered essential because our bodies either don't produce adequate amounts or do not produce them at all so we must get them from our diets or supplements.

This is a large number of nutrients to track in your daily diet. My strategy of focusing on nutrient-dense foods eliminates the need to track individual nutrients by simply eating foods that provide them at healthy levels. As you will see in Section V, you can achieve almost all the daily recommended micronutrient levels by following this strategy.[114] [115]

I have also included a brief chapter on phytonutrients at the end of this section. These nutrients are produced by plants and are a relatively new area of nutrition. Studies show that several phytonutrients have antioxidant, antimicrobial, anti-inflammatory, and anticancer properties. Since the science on these nutrients is still developing, this chapter is meant to be purely educational and does not include a dietary strategy.

Micronutrient measurement: As background, micronutrients are usually measured in milligrams (mg) equal to 1,000th of a gram or micrograms (mcg) equal to 1 millionth of a gram. Very small amounts!

You will sometimes see the measurement term "ug" used for certain micronutrients. This is an equivalent measure to micrograms (i.e., 1 mcg = 1 ug). You may also see the term "IU," sometimes used for measurement of certain vitamins. Many supplements now convert IUs to milligrams on their labels.

Let's move on now to Chapter 8, which describes the micronutrients most Americans struggle to get in adequate amounts.

Micronutrient Inadequacies and Priorities

The U.S. FNB has developed daily recommendations (DRIs) for most essential micronutrients. These recommendations are accepted by credible nutrition information sources. I use these as nutritional benchmarks for all food and meal analyses in Sections IV and V.

Unfortunately, many studies show that Americans don't achieve these recommended daily levels. Two terms are used to describe this nutrient shortfall: nutrient deficiency and nutrient inadequacy. Although these terms are often used inter-changeably, they are quite different.

A **micronutrient deficiency** is defined as having severely reduced levels of one or more nutrients. This causes major health issues, which become apparent quickly and can result in the body being unable to perform one or more important functions. Fortunately, such micronutrient deficiencies are rare in the U.S.

A **micronutrient inadequacy** occurs when intake levels are consistently below a nutrient's DRI. The health consequences of micronutrient inadequacies can be difficult to identify, as symptoms may not appear for several years or decades. However, many studies indicate that inadequacies of certain micronutrients increase the risk of several chronic conditions, including cancer, cardiovascular disease, type 2 diabetes, osteoporosis, and eye diseases. Micronutrient inadequacies may also suppress our immune system and increase the risk of impaired brain function.

Micronutrient Inadequacies in the U.S.

So, which micronutrients have inadequacies in the U.S.? The best available source for this information is a bi-annual U.S. nutritional survey called the National Health and Nutrition Examination Survey (NHANES). These surveys have been conducted by the CDC over the past several decades.

The NHANES work is considered one of the most complete and respected nutritional data sets in the world. It includes not just food intake surveys, but also interviews, physical examinations, and biomarker tests (e.g., blood and urine tests) for adult and child participants.[116]

Many studies have been carried out on the NHANES survey data. I selected one specific study for my research because it analyzed NHANES data over a long time period (2005–2016), giving it more credibility.

This study found many vitamins and minerals with high inadequacy rates among U.S. adults. Vitamins D (95%), E

(84%), C (46%), A (45%), and K (45%) were the highest. As for minerals, magnesium (53%), calcium (43%), and zinc (15%) were the highest. Also, B9 folate (12%) and B6 pantothenic acid (11%) had double digit inadequacy rates.

Even when supplements were considered, inadequacy rates were not reduced significantly. Other studies of NHANES data have found similar inadequacy rates among these same micronutrients.

Some of these studies have reported even higher inadequacy rates among the elderly for zinc as well as vitamin B12. More recent studies have shown that less than 45% of the U.S. elderly population consumes adequate levels of zinc and may have deficiency rates as high as 40%. One study found a B12 deficiency rate of 10–15% among the elderly. [117] [118] [119]

Micronutrient Dietary Priorities

Given these findings, we need to prioritize certain micronutrients in our diets to ensure we get recommended daily levels. The health risks of these inadequacies are far too great.

In addition to these micronutrients, we should also prioritize potassium, choline, and iron for the following reasons:

- **Potassium** was not included in this NHANES study, but other studies show U.S. adults have inadequacy rates up to 50%. This important mineral supports many health functions and has a critical role in lowering blood pressure.[120]

- **Choline** is believed to have a very high inadequacy rate, with some studies showing over 90%. This nutrient is important for brain health.[121]
- **Iron** has an inadequacy rate relatively high among women (pre-menopausal). One study found an iron deficiency rate especially high among adolescent women at approximately 40%. This results in a significant health risk for these women.[122]

Lastly, **sodium** should be prioritized in our diets not as a result of an inadequacy, but rather its significant over-consumption in the U.S. This is a major cause of high blood pressure and is associated with several cardiovascular diseases. Sodium should be limited in your diet. [123]

I realize this is a large number of nutrients to prioritize, but as you will see below, all of these micronutrients have key roles in ensuring good health. If I were to ask you whether your heart, brain, or lungs are more important for your health, how would you answer? My guess is you would say I need all of these to work well for my good health. Well, you need all of these micronutrients consistently at recommended levels for good health as well.

This is what makes establishing a healthy diet so difficult. It is also why I recommend you focus your daily diet on consuming the most nutritious foods to get these micronutrients. This is a much easier approach than nutrient counting.

In the next two chapters, I describe each priority micro-nutrient's DRI, UL (daily upper limit), health purpose and the foods containing healthy levels. You do not have to memorize this information; rather, think of it as an opportunity to gain a broader understanding of this area of nutrition.

The later book sections will describe the best foods and meals to reach adequate daily levels.

CHAPTER 9

Vitamins

Vitamins fall into two categories: fat-soluble or water-soluble. Vitamins A, D, E, and K are fat-soluble. Excess amounts of fat-soluble vitamins are stored in our livers and fat cells. It is thought that these vitamins are stored for a few days to several months, depending on the vitamin.

Water-soluble vitamins are not stored, with excess amounts excreted daily, usually through urine. Vitamins C and the Bs are water-soluble. These vitamins should be consumed every day to avoid inadequacies. The exception is vitamin B12, which is stored in the liver.

Priority Vitamins

Vitamin C: DRI of 75 mg/day for adult females and 90 mg/day for adult males. UL of 2,000 mg/day.

Vitamin C has a high inadequacy rate of nearly 50%. We need to take in adequate levels of this vitamin daily.

A powerful antioxidant, Vitamin C's health benefits include collagen production and wound healing. This helps keep skin, cartilage, and blood vessel cells healthy. In addition, it supports absorption of non-heme iron (plant-based) and regeneration (recreation) of other antioxidants such as vitamin E and glutathione, a strong antioxidant produced by the body.

Vitamin C further supports metabolic functions for energy production and immune health, especially with the production of white blood cells for fighting infections.

DYK

Vitamin C can be depleted during severe infections, so get extra vitamin C when you have a bad cold!

There are several healthy fruit and vegetable options to achieve the DRI for this vitamin. I get my recommended levels of vitamin C by regularly consuming citrus fruits, berries, sweet peppers, and broccoli. Sweet and baked potatoes and avocados are also great sources for this nutrient.

B vitamins: DRIs and ULs for B vitamins vary by each type and are summarized below:

B VITAMIN	DRI ADULT FEMALE	DRI ADULT MALE	UL
Thiamin (B1)	1.1 mg	1.2 mg	None
Riboflavin (B2)	1.1 mg	1.3 mg	None
Niacin (B3)	14 mg	16 mg	30 mg
Pantothenic acid (B5)	5 mg (AI)	5 mg (AI)	None
Pyridoxine (B6)	1.3 mg	1.3 mg	100 mg
Folate (B9)	400 mcg	400 mcg	1000 mcg
Cobalamins (B12)	2.4 mcg	2.4 mcg	None

B vitamins are often referred to as B complex. These vitamins are also water-soluble and need to be replenished in our bodies daily (except B12). Most are considered antioxidants or have antioxidant-like properties.

B vitamins support many important metabolic functions. These include converting food into energy, building cell DNA, transporting nutrients throughout the body, creating new red blood cells, and maintaining healthy cells in our skin, brains, and other body tissues.

Vitamins B6, B9 (known as folate), and B12 are particularly important for breaking down and lowering an enzyme called homocysteine. High levels of homocysteine are associated with chronic inflammation and increased risk of blood clots, cardio-vascular disease, osteoporosis, and dementia.

Most B vitamins are found in healthy amounts in several animal and plant foods. Unfortunately, a few are only present in a small number of foods.

As an example, B12 is not naturally found in plant foods, but is in many animal foods at healthy levels. Therefore, vegetarians can struggle to get adequate levels of this nutrient. Conversely, B9 is found in very few animal foods and usually only at moderate levels. Fortunately, you can get plenty of B9 from plant foods.

In the next few chapters, I identify foods that contain healthy levels of B vitamins. If you eat a balanced diet full of these fresh animal and whole plant foods, then you will be able to meet the daily B complex recommendations.

If you have dietary restrictions, then a supplement may be warranted. Consult your physician before taking a B vitamin supplement to discuss the right levels for you.

Vitamin D: DRI of 15 micrograms (or 600 IU) for adults ages 18–70 years. UL of 100 mcg (or 4000 IU).

Vitamin D has the highest micronutrient inadequacy rate for U.S. adults at approximately 95%. However, it is fat-soluble, meaning excess amounts are stored by the body for future needs. Therefore, there is more daily dietary flexibility with this micronutrient.

The high inadequacy rate is due in part to the fact that so few foods contain this important vitamin. It's found at healthy levels only in a few types of fish and fortified foods.

In addition to our diets, we get vitamin D from sunlight on our skin. In fact, sunlight is our primary source of vitamin D. The high inadequacy rate is thus also the result of many of us not getting outside as much as our ancestors.

Adequate levels of vitamin D are critical for good bone health, as it helps our bodies absorb and maintain healthy levels of calcium and phosphorus. Note that adequate levels of magnesium are needed to support vitamin D levels, as magnesium is needed for its metabolism.

Vitamin D is also believed to support our immune system and reduce inflammation and depression. Though not considered an antioxidant, it has many of the same properties as one.

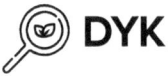

DYK

Studies show that our bodies may store vitamin D for up to several months. These stores may be used when there is low access to sun, such as during the winter months.

The best strategy to achieve the vitamin D DRI is to get outside in the sun regularly. While there are concerns about sun exposure damaging skin, studies show that it may only take 15–30 minutes to achieve DRI levels. Also, make sure to regularly consume fatty fish or fortified foods. These fish are identified in the next section.

If you don't get outside regularly and are not a fan of fish, consider taking a vitamin D supplement. Credible health information sources recommend supplements of between 15–50 mcg (or 600–2,000 IU). Vitamin D3 appears to be the most effective form of supplement.

To get adequate levels of vitamin D, I consume fatty fish typically twice a week. I also get outside quite a bit and wear sunscreen when I'm out for periods over 15–20 minutes. When I'm not getting outside often or in the cold winter months, I take a supplement. My supplement contains levels above the UL, so I cut the pills in quarters to get my supplement down to DRI levels.

Be careful not to overdo it with vitamin D supplements. While rare, excess amounts of vitamin D can be toxic by increasing your calcium absorption to harmful levels. This is called hypercalcemia which may cause calcium buildup in arteries and kidney stones.

Vitamin E: DRI of 15 milligrams/day for adults and adolescents over age 14 years. UL of 1,000 mg/day.

Vitamin E is another nutrient with a high inadequacy rate in the U.S. It is a powerful antioxidant and a fat-soluble vitamin.

Studies show vitamin E supports immune system function and may reduce the risk of contracting upper respiratory tract viral infections, especially for the elderly and smokers. It has also been associated with good eye, skin, and brain health.

With its high inadequacy rate, vitamin E is an important micronutrient to focus on in your diet. There are a few animal foods with moderate to high levels and several plant foods and oils with healthy amounts.

I get my daily vitamin E from almonds in my morning oatmeal, sunflower seeds in my lunch smoothie, and an occasional snack of peanuts. I also regularly eat salmon, avocados, and tomato-based pasta sauces, all good sources for this nutrient.

If you decide to take a supplement, be careful about taking too much vitamin E and consult with your physician. High supplement doses above the UL may increase the risk of stroke and interrupt blood coagulation for individuals on blood thinners. It has also been linked to an increased risk of prostate cancer. However, more research is needed to verify these findings.

Vitamin A: DRI of 700 micrograms/day for adult females and 900 mcg/day for adult males. UL of 3,000 mcg/day.

Vitamin A's inadequacy rate is relatively high at 45%.

Another important antioxidant, vitamin A comes in two dietary forms: preformed A and provitamin A. The preformed version comes from animal foods, while provitamin A comes from plant foods. Beta carotene is a phytonutrient carotenoid in primarily plant foods that converts into vitamin A in the body.

Vitamin A promotes white blood cell growth and function, which supports our immune systems. It has also been found to inhibit inflammation and has a role in cell growth and maintenance. Although studies have not proven that vitamin A plays a key role in supporting eye health, many foods high in beta-carotene are also high in the carotenoids lutein and zeaxanthin, which have been shown to support eye health.

There are a few animal foods that have high levels of vitamin A. Several plant foods contain moderate to high levels of it, notably certain root vegetables. The foods highest in vitamin A are described later in the book.

Be careful about taking high supplement doses of vitamin A as they are associated with harmful health effects. In particular, if you are pregnant, then please consult your physician before taking a vitamin A supplement, as high doses are associated with birth defects.

Vitamin K: DRI of 90 micrograms/day for adult females and 120 mcg for adult males. No UL.

Vitamin K is the least studied and understood vitamin. It comes in two forms: Vitamin K1, phylloquinone, that we get from plant foods, while Vitamin K2, menaquinone, is found in modest amounts in animal and fermented foods.

Studies show that vitamin K supports blood coagulation (K1) and bone health (K2). These studies link dietary vitamin K2 to a reduced risk of osteoporosis and lower fracture rates for women.

K1 intake inadequacy rates are approximately 45% for adult Americans. It is metabolized quickly by our bodies and eliminated through waste. This may increase the possibility of vitamin K1 inadequacies, but research shows when the body is low in this nutrient it recycles used vitamin K.

To minimize any potential inadequacies, make sure you regularly consume foods with vitamin K in your diet. I highlight these foods in subsequent chapters.

Lastly, there is no established UL for vitamin K, as the risk of toxicity from excessive amounts is believed to be low.

Choline: DRI of 425 milligrams for adult females and 550 mg for adult males. UL of 3,500 mg for all adults.

Choline is an essential nutrient that is neither a vitamin nor a mineral. It was discovered and established as an essential nutrient in 1998. The liver makes small amounts of choline, but the rest must come from our diet.

Choline supports the brain and nervous system by regulating memory, mood, and brain development and function. New studies show that having low levels of choline may increase the risk of Alzheimer's.

Choline is also believed to support muscle control, regular heartbeat, formation of cell membranes, DNA synthesis, and liver health, as well as fat metabolism by removing cholesterol from the liver.

It is estimated that 90% of Americans do not take in the DRI for choline. The good news is that you can get adequate choline levels through a balanced diet of several different animal foods, described in the following chapters. Very few plant foods contain healthy levels.

Fatty fish (salmon, tuna, etc.), eggs, and lean beef are all great sources of choline. I consume these foods regularly to get this critical nutrient. Eggs are particularly high in choline.

📖 Vitamins Facts Break

➤ *Few animal foods have healthy levels of vitamin C, but a typical serving of cooked broccoli, cooked kale, strawberries, or red sweet peppers provide over 100% of the DRI.*

➤ *Consuming foods with unsaturated fats at the same time or day as fat-soluble vitamin foods improves absorption of these vitamins. Examples of such unsaturated fats foods include nuts, fatty fish, avocados, and olive oil.*

➤ *The best sources for vitamin D are salmon and farmed rainbow trout, which contain over 100% of the DRI.*

➤ *Water-soluble vitamins (C and the Bs) in vegetables are often reduced during cooking. These nutrients are lost at highest levels with boiling and poaching cooking methods. Sauteing and stir frying are among the best for retaining these vitamins.*

Additional sources used for vitamins description: [124] [125] [126] [127] [128] [129] [130] [131] [132] [133] [134] [135] [136] [137] [138] [139] [140]

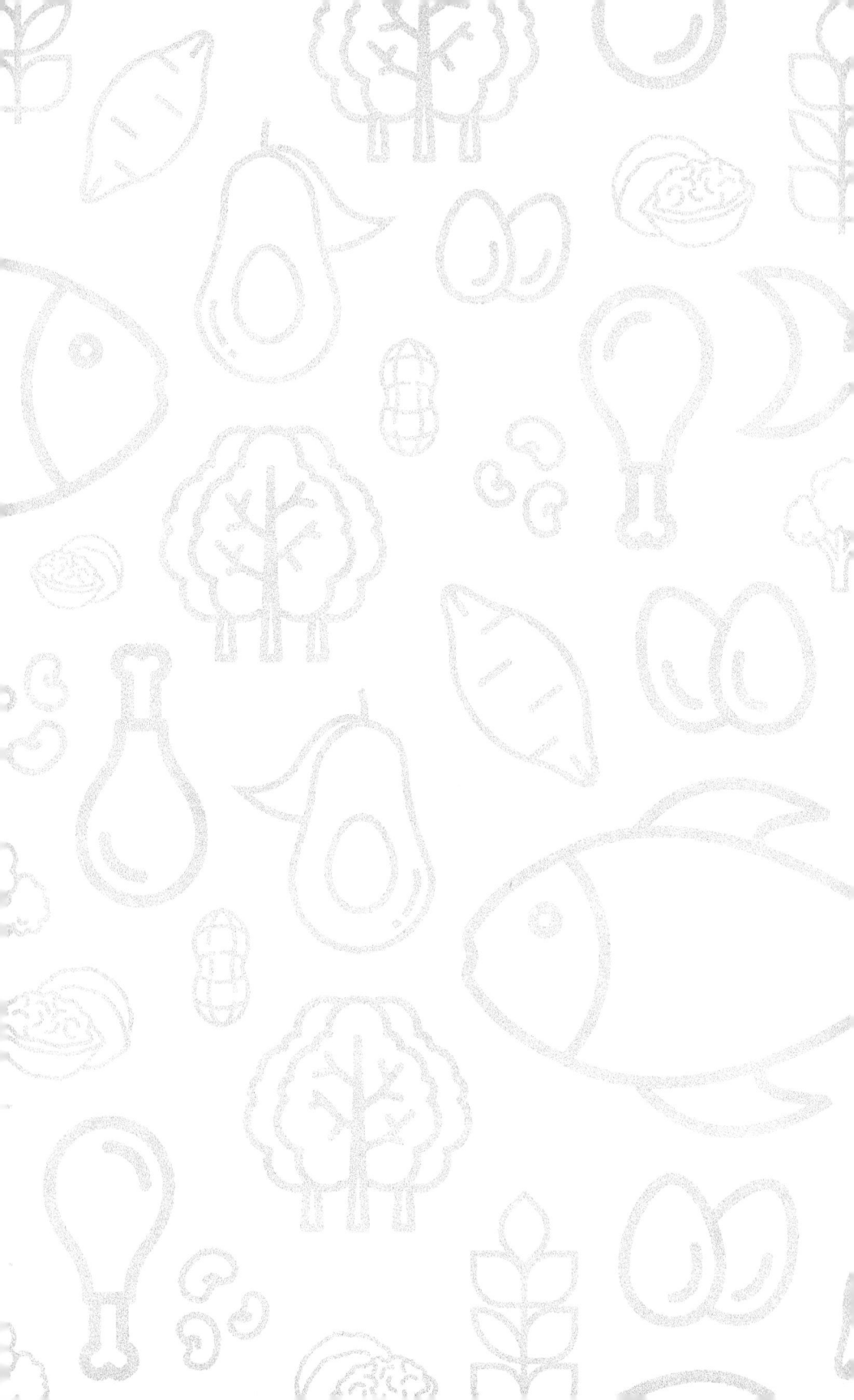

CHAPTER 10

Minerals

Minerals are divided into two categories: major and trace. You need to consume higher amounts of major minerals than trace for good health. Excess minerals are stored in our bones, muscles, livers, and other tissues. It is not well understood how long these nutrients are stored.

Major minerals include calcium, magnesium, sodium, potassium, chloride, phosphorus, and sulfur. Trace minerals include iron, zinc, manganese, selenium, copper, fluoride, and iodine.

Priority Minerals

Zinc: DRI of 8 mg for adult females and 11 mg for adult males. UL of 40 mg/day.

Unlike other minerals, our bodies don't store zinc in significant amounts. Therefore, it needs to be replenished regularly in our diets.

An antioxidant, zinc supports several important health areas related to cellular metabolism. It facilitates hundreds of enzyme chemical reactions important for energy levels, brain health and function, immune function, production of important proteins, healthy DNA, cellular growth, wound healing, and skin health.

Zinc is also believed to help reduce the duration of respiratory infections, improve blood sugar levels, reduce the risk of type 2 diabetes, and decrease levels of LDL cholesterol and triglycerides.

Zinc inadequacies are thought to be uncommon in healthy adults, likely due to its availability at moderate to high levels in several foods, especially animal foods. The exception is elderly populations, where there are high rates of zinc inadequacies and deficiencies.

If you are a vegetarian, legumes, tree nuts, peanuts, whole grains, and seeds are your best sources for this key nutrient. Unfortunately, none of these plant foods contain high levels (nor do eggs or cheese). If you are concerned about your daily zinc intake, you may want to consider taking a supplement and should discuss this with your physician.

If you do regularly take a zinc supplement, it is recommended that you stay within the 15–30 mg per day range. Do not exceed the UL of 40mg per day, which increases the risks of certain health issues.

Calcium: DRI of 1,000 milligrams/day for adult females up to age 50 and adult males up to age 70. Above these ages, DRI increases to 1,200 mg. UL of 2,500 mg/day for all adults up to age 50 and up to 2,000 mg for those over 50.

Calcium is the most abundant mineral in our bodies and, along with phosphorus, makes up much of our bone and teeth structure. Our bones are constantly growing and repairing to maintain good health, and calcium is critical to this process.

Adequate calcium is needed to reduce the risks of osteopenia (reduction in bone density) and osteoporosis. Calcium is also critical for maintaining the structure of brain cells, regulating brain function, and supporting blood flow.

Calcium is among several major minerals considered electrolytes. Magnesium, sodium, potassium, chloride, and phosphate are the others. Electrolytes support fluid balance, pH balance, the transport of nutrients into and waste out of cells, muscle and nerve function, normal heart rate rhythm, and stable blood pressure.

Unfortunately, there is a relatively high incidence of inadequate intake of this important mineral among U.S. adults at over 40%. This is likely the result of so few foods containing healthy amounts. In the U.S., we get approximately 70% of calcium from dairy products. Given that approximately 90 million American adults have issues digesting the lactose in dairy (intolerance and malabsorption), it is not surprising that inadequacy rates are so high.

In addition, calcium's overall digestive absorption rate is relatively low compared to other nutrients, especially among the elderly. This is due to nutrient absorption decreasing as we age. It also may be the result of the elderly tending to have lower levels of vitamin D, which is critical for maintaining healthy calcium levels.

This is my most difficult mineral to reach at daily recommended levels. I do consume moderate amounts of Greek yogurt and kefir in my morning oatmeal, and regularly eat canned fish, kale, and 100% whole-wheat bread, which typically have moderate levels. To date, my blood test panel has shown normal levels of calcium, but if this starts to go lower then I will consider increasing my dairy intake or taking a supplement.

You may want to consider a supplement if you are lactose intolerant, elderly, a vegan, or have low blood levels of calcium. Be careful not to take a supplement with levels far above the UL. Doing so may pose serious health risks. You may want to discuss taking a supplement with your physician before starting.

Magnesium: DRI for adults over age 30, 320 mg for females and 420 mg for males. Slightly lower for adults under age 30. UL for supplements is 350 mg/day. There is no UL for magnesium in foods.

Magnesium is another important mineral to our health and unfortunately over half of all U.S. adults have inadequate intake.

Magnesium supports enzyme reactions that regulate blood pressure, produce energy from carbohydrates and fats, make proteins and DNA, transport potassium and calcium into/out of cells, and regulate blood glucose levels. Most type 2 diabetics have low magnesium levels.

Magnesium is another electrolyte and offers all the electrolyte health benefits described under calcium. Most magnesium is stored in our bones, with the remainder in muscles or other soft tissue. It also supports the structural development of bones.

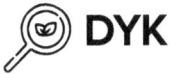

DYK

Magnesium helps convert vitamin D to its active form. This is the reason adequate levels of magnesium, vitamin D, calcium, and phosphorus are all interrelated for good bone health.

Studies have found an association between low levels of magnesium and low glutathione levels (a powerful antioxidant made by the body). These low levels are also related to high oxidative stress and metabolic syndrome. These health issues are described in more detail in Section I.

Further, magnesium has been shown to be effective in reducing the incidence of acute migraine headaches and is endorsed as a treatment by the American Academy of Neurology and the American Headache Society.

Magnesium is found in several animal and plant foods in moderate to high levels and these are identified in the next two sections.

🏅 Pro Move

Pumpkin seeds, cacao powder (less processed version of cocoa), and chia seeds are all high in magnesium. Try adding a couple of tablespoons of these to your morning oatmeal, to smoothies, or to meal recipes.

The UL for magnesium supplements (and medicines) is low compared to the DRI because even moderate doses can cause gastrointestinal issues. Foods high in magnesium have not been found to cause these issues.

Lastly, taking high levels of vitamin D supplements above the UL have been shown to lower magnesium levels.

Sodium: DRI of 1.5 grams for all adults. UL of 2.3 grams (approximately 1 teaspoon of salt).

Sodium is on this list not for inadequate intake, but rather for excessive intake. It is an electrolyte, so it's an important mineral to have in your diet, but not at levels above the UL.

Unfortunately, Americans consume far too much sodium. The FDA states that the average American takes in approximately 3.4 grams of sodium per day, more than twice the DRI and nearly 50% above the UL. The FDA strongly recommends that all Americans monitor and reduce their sodium intake.

High sodium consumption increases blood pressure. High blood pressure increases the risk of several cardiovascular diseases including heart attacks and stroke. It also increases the risk of other health issues such as kidney disease and vision problems. Further, certain high-sodium foods can increase the risk of gastric cancer.

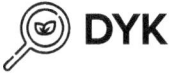

DYK

High blood pressure is a chronic condition that is now at epidemic levels in the U.S. Half of the adult population, or over 120 million Americans, have hypertension.

In addition, studies show that high sodium levels increase the loss of calcium through urine. This can lower bone mineral density and increase the risk of osteoporosis. This health risk is highest among the elderly, especially women.

Except for some seafoods, unprocessed animal and plant foods naturally have low levels of sodium. This means that we get our high sodium either from processed foods, restaurant meals, or the salt we put in our food. Focus on limiting daily sodium to no more than the UL.

It is easy to go over the UL for sodium, so reducing salt intake takes discipline, especially if you are used to adding it to your food. Please try to lower amounts in your diet for extended periods of time. You may find that you become more sensitive to it and as a result don't need high levels to improve the taste of your food. At restaurants, try asking for low-sodium menu options when available.

🏅 Pro Move

Try substituting flavor enhancers for salt in meals. Garlic, spices, and citrus juices are all great options. Avoid processed meats that are cured, salted, or smoked and often high in sodium. Lastly, get healthy levels of potassium in your diet or try a salt substitute that contains potassium. This helps reduce sodium in the body (see below).

To determine how much sodium is in your grocery store foods, check the nutrition facts labels. The sodium content will be presented in mg and as a percentage of daily value (for sodium this equals the UL).

Potassium: DRI of 2.6 grams for adult women per day and 3.4 grams for adult men. No UL, as normal kidney function eliminates excess potassium.

Potassium is another electrolyte with all the health benefits stated above.

Another important potassium health benefit is that it helps offset the risks associated with the overconsumption of sodium. Several studies show that potassium helps our bodies remove excess sodium, relaxes blood vessels, and improves cardiovascular health.

The AHA and the U.S. National Academy of Science both endorse diets high in potassium and low in sodium to help reduce the risk of high blood pressure and stroke. In fact, the

AHA recommends that Americans with high blood pressure take in 3.5 to 5 grams daily.

Studies have also shown that high potassium intake is linked to healthy brain function and cognitive health. It further reduces the risk of kidney stones and is believed to help prevent calcium loss from our bones.

Other studies have found an association between low levels of potassium and increased blood glucose levels and type 2 diabetes.

Unfortunately, the U.S. adult population's intake of potassium has an inadequacy rate up to 50%, with some studies showing even higher rates.

Potassium is found in several plant and animal foods, but mostly at only moderate levels. I get my potassium from both animal and plant sources. These include fresh and canned fatty fish, chicken, red meat, avocados, peanuts, broccoli, and tomato-based pasta sauce. Sweet and baked potatoes and legumes are also healthy sources for this important mineral. These foods are all described in more detail in Section IV.

Iron: DRI of 18 mg for adult females and 8 mg for adult males. Over age 50, the female DRI drops to 8 mg. UL of 45 mg for all ages 14 and over.

Most iron in the body is contained in hemoglobin, a protein found in red blood cells. Iron binds to oxygen molecules which in turn bind to the hemoglobin. In this form, the oxygen is ready to be transported in our blood from the lungs to the cells in our brains, muscles, and other tissues.

Iron is also an important nutrient for cell growth, energy production, immune system support, neurological development, and the formation of hormones and tissues.

While it is believed that overall iron inadequacy rates are low in the U.S., a recent study found as many as 15% of all adult Americans suffer from an iron deficiency. Young women between the ages 12–21 have a nearly 40% deficiency rate.

Iron deficiency can result in anemia, a low level of healthy red blood cells with hemoglobin. This is a serious health issue. Anemia can affect brain focus, muscle performance, and stamina, and increase the risk of infections.

You may have noticed from the DRIs listed above that the female recommendation for iron is 2.5 times that for males. Menstruating women and pregnant women, in particular, should be intentional in their diet to ensure they get adequate levels of iron.

🎖 Pro Move

Heme iron (from animals) is absorbed well by our bodies, but non-heme iron from plant foods is not. Vitamin C and heme iron are both believed to improve non-heme iron absorption when consumed at the same meal. So, for your next meal, add some meat or foods high in vitamin C to your plant foods' iron to absorb it at higher levels.

Most animal foods have at least moderate amounts of iron, except dairy. Most red meats and oysters are the highest sources. Chicken, fatty fish, clams and eggs have moderate levels for women.

Among the best plant sources are legumes, especially soybeans, whole wheat bread and quinoa, baked potatoes, tomato sauce, spinach, chia and pumpkin seeds, and cacao powder. Most of these foods have iron at moderate levels for women.

If you are considering a supplement, it is best not to exceed the UL. You should discuss your iron supplement with your physician before taking one.

📖 Supplements Facts Break

→ *When consuming a well-balanced diet full of whole, unprocessed animal and plant foods, it is usually not necessary to take a multi-vitamin.*

→ *If you believe you are low in certain nutrients and can't get them from your food, consider taking a nutrient-specific supplement. Given that some supplements interact poorly with certain medications, it is best to discuss your supplement decisions with your doctor before taking.*

→ *Supplements are not as highly regulated as food. Be careful, as some provide nutrients at amounts well above their UL. Choose supplements below the UL or cut them into halves or quarters to stay within healthy levels.*

Additional sources used for minerals description: [141] [142] [143] [144] [145] [146] [147] [148] [149] [150] [151]

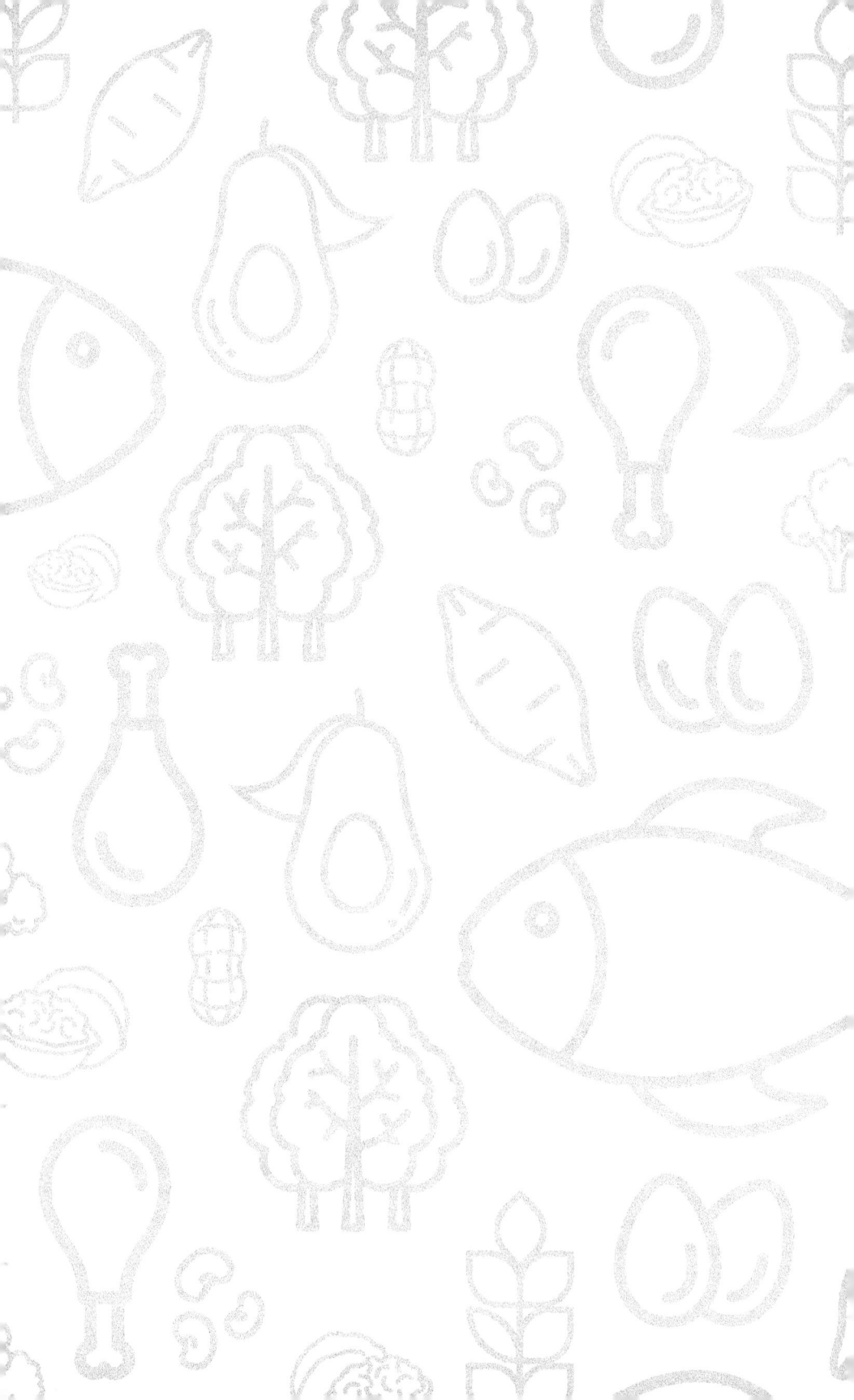

CHAPTER 11

Phytonutrients

Phytonutrients, also called phytochemicals or polyphenols, are a new nutritional area that has emerged over the last few decades. They are primarily found in plants and highly concentrated in plant peels, skins, and seeds.

Phytonutrients are natural chemicals and compounds produced by all plants. They protect the plants against viruses, bacteria, fungi, insects, and UV light. Certain drinks like coffee and tea are rich in phytonutrients.

The science on phytonutrients is still evolving. Consequently, there are no specific daily intake recommendations from the FNB or any other U.S. health agency. As a result, this book gives no specific intake recommendations on levels of phytonutrients. However, given their significant potential health benefits, I do want to provide some information about them.

Studies show these nutrients have antioxidant, antimicrobial, anti-inflammatory, and anticancer properties. Phytonutrients have several potential health benefits, including improved brain cognition; stress reduction; better sleep; and improved immune, digestive, bone, joint, and cardiovascular health.

You may already be using certain phytonutrient products. For example, athletes use them to improve performance and recovery (e.g., anthocyanins in tart cherry juice), while some people use them as topical creams to reduce wrinkles and increase collagen production (flavonoids, beta-carotene, lycopene, and lutein).

There are over 10,000 phytonutrients identified, and the number is growing. Below, I list well-known phytonutrients with credible science defining their health benefits. Also, note that there are various classifications used for phytonutrients, which can vary greatly. I used one from an NIH-published study.

All of these phytonutrients are contained in the foods I recommend in the remaining book sections. In the descriptions below, I have included a table showing each major phytonutrient's classes and subclasses (if applicable) and the foods believed to include significant amounts.

Major Phytonutrients

Flavonoids are the most studied phytonutrient. They are high in antioxidants and are believed to provide immune protection from various toxins. There are many different flavonoids and subclasses, and as a group they have shown anticancer, antibacterial, antiviral, and antifungal properties. Flavonoids are believed to support cardiovascular, blood sugar, and inflammation health, and are also associated with the reduction of neurodegenerative diseases.

FLAVONOLS Subclasses: quercetin, kaempferol, myricetin, and isorhamnetin	**Foods:** Onions, ancho and hot chili peppers, kale, spinach, purple sweet potatoes, blueberries, cherries, chia seeds, ginger, and black tea.
FLAVONES Subclasses: apigenin and luteolin	**Foods:** Celery, parsley, peppermint, and thyme.
FLAVON-3-OLS Subclasses: catechins, epicatechins, theaflavins, thiouridines, and epigallo-catechins (and others)	**Foods:** Cacao products, blueberries, blackberries, black grapes, plums, white peaches, sweet cherries, apples (with skin), apricots, soybeans, pecans, and black/green/white tea.
FLAVANONES Subclasses: hesperidin, naringenin, eriodyctiol, and pinostrobin	**Foods:** Citrus fruits like oranges, grapefruits, tangerines, lemons, and limes.
ANTHOCYANIDINS/ ANTHOCYANIN Subclasses: cyanidin, delphinidin, malvidin, pelargonidin, peonidin, and petunidin	**Foods:** Blueberries, blackberries, raspberries, strawberries, sweet cherries, concord and red grapes, plums, apples (with skin), pears (with skin), red cabbage, pecans, black beans, and black-eyed peas.

Carotenoids act as antioxidants and anti-inflammatories. There are more than 600 carotenoids. The most well-known are beta-carotene, lycopene, lutein, and zeaxanthin. Beta-carotene converts to vitamin A and has all the same health benefits.

Lycopene protects against colorectal, breast, and prostate cancers. Some studies show lycopene also reduces the risk of heart disease, type 2 diabetes, and cognitive decline, and further protects skin against sunburn.

Lutein and zeaxanthin help lower the risk of cataracts and age-related macular degeneration. Studies also show an association with good heart and bone health, cognitive function, and lower cancer risk.

Beta-carotene	Foods: Sweet potatoes, pumpkin, carrots, kale, spinach, and cooked broccoli.
Lycopene	Foods: Tomatoes, grapefruit, and watermelon. Tomato's lycopene increases and absorbs better when cooked. Red pasta and stewed tomatoes are good examples. Sundried tomatoes also have high levels.
Lutein and zeaxanthin	Foods: Spinach, kale, green peas, Brussel sprouts, broccoli, and parsley. They are also found in pistachios, eggs with yolk, avocado, quinoa, and 100% whole wheat.

Organosulfur compounds are found in alliaceous and cruciferous vegetables. Studies show that these plant-based sulfur compounds are antioxidants that support our immune systems, are antiviral, reduce inflammation, and possibly improve bone health.

Alliaceous plants have sulfuric compounds believed to help prevent certain cancers, including prostate and potentially breast cancer.

Cruciferous vegetables contain a compound named glucosinolates. Studies show its potential health benefits include reducing inflammation and lowering the risk of certain cancers and cardiovascular disease.

Alliaceous plants	Foods: Garlic, onions, shallots, leeks, scallions, and chives.
Cruciferous plants	Foods: Broccoli, Brussel sprouts, kale, cabbage, cauliflower, arugula, radish, and turnips.

Phenolic Acids have antioxidant, anti-inflammatory, antimicrobial, and antimutagenic (reduces mutations in DNA) properties. They are believed to protect against health risks related to cardiovascular disease, neurodegenerative disease, cancer, and diabetes. Some of the most studied phenolic acids include ellagic, vanillic, syringic, and cinnamic.

Ellagic acid	**Foods:** Blackberries, strawberries, raspberries, pomegranates, red grapes, walnuts, pistachios, cashews, pecans, apples, and green tea.
Vanillic and syringic acid	**Foods:** Dried and fresh dates, cranberries, olives, grapefruits, dried and fresh sage, dried sweet basil, green tea, whole grains, walnuts, grapes, and pumpkins.
Cinnamic acid	**Foods:** Coffee, cinnamon, tea, cocoa, citrus fruits, sweet potatoes, artichokes, grapes, peanuts, walnuts, pecans, celery, basil, cruciferous vegetables, spinach, garlic, quinoa, 100% whole wheat, and whole-grain rice.

Phytoestrogens provide estrogen-like nutrients that exhibit anti-inflammatory, antioxidant, and anticancer properties. Phytoestrogens support our immune systems and are believed to support reproductive, heart, bone, immune, and skin health. They are also associated with a reduced risk of certain cancers, liver disease, diabetes, cognitive decline, and obesity. Three of the major categories of phytoestrogens are isoflavones, lignans, and resveratrol.

Isoflavones	**Foods:** Soybeans, fermented soy products like miso and tempeh, tofu, and food products with soy protein powder.
Lignans	**Foods:** Flax seeds and sesame seeds/oil contain very high amounts. Lesser amounts in kale, broccoli, Brussel sprouts, white cabbage, green beans, green peppers, apricots, pears, and cashews.
Resveratrol	**Foods:** Red grapes, sweet potatoes, walnuts, peanuts (with skin), oats, red apples, peaches, pears, oranges, tangerines, and grapefruits.

Additional sources used for phytonutrients description: [152] [153] [154] [155] [156] [157] [158] [159] [160] [161] [162] [163] [164] [165] [166] [167] [168] [169] [170] [171] [172]

SECTION III KEY TAKEAWAYS

- **Micronutrient dietary goal:** Regularly consume foods and meals that achieve micronutrient DRIs. Priority micronutrients are ones of which Americans have the highest inadequacy levels and pose significant health risks as a result. These include all vitamins, and the minerals calcium, magnesium, potassium, zinc, iron, and choline. Many of these nutrients are also antioxidants that protect the body against oxidative stress.

- **Sodium:** Monitor your sodium intake and try to stay under the daily UL of 2.3g. Half of the U.S. adult population has high blood pressure, which is a significant health risk, and high sodium intake is a leading cause. Read the nutrition facts labels on your foods and focus on those with low sodium levels. Also, consume the daily recommended levels of potassium as this mineral helps to eliminate excess sodium from the body.

- **Supplements:** When taking micronutrient supplements, try not to exceed the UL. Several micronutrients can cause adverse health effects when taken at levels above the UL. Also, supplements can interact poorly with some medications. Discuss your supplement intake with your physician, especially if you are on any medications.

- **Phytonutrients:** This relatively new nutritional area needs more research. There are no daily dietary phytonutrient intake recommendations. That said, the studies performed to date show that these nutrients may offer several important health benefits. The most studied phytonutrients are contained in the foods recommended in this book.

SECTION IV

Nutrient-Dense and Nutritious Foods

Now we get to the fun stuff: the food!

The previous sections have provided a fundamental understanding of nutrition, its importance to our health, and how inadequate intake levels can harm our health. Now, I want to begin to define how my approach to a nutrient-dense diet will ensure that you get all the nutrition your body needs.

The first step is to identify and describe the most nutritious foods available to us. That's what this section is all about. Chapter 12 defines my approach for evaluating these foods' nutrient content. The following three chapters detail specific nutritious foods that we should have in our diets.

The last chapter in this section (Chapter 16) identifies the ten most nutritious foods and a few others that nearly made this list. These are the foods that I recommend be in your diet weekly, if not daily. This chapter provides further details by showing each food's specific levels of macro and micronutrients.

All these chapters will help establish the groundwork for Section V, in which I provide example meals using the nutritious foods described in this section. Consistently consuming these or similar meals will provide you with almost full daily nutrition.

If you've read the previous sections of the book, I hope you've learned some valuable nutritional information. For those of you who have not read sections I–III, you can consult the key takeaways at the end of each one. Further, before I dive into the specific foods, you may want to read the explanations below. These will help you understand certain terms used throughout sections IV and V.

Daily U.S. macro and micronutrient recommendations are made by the U.S. Food and Nutrition Board (FNB). The FNB establishes Dietary Reference Intakes (DRIs). There are three primary DRI levels given. The levels are described as:

- Recommended Dietary Allowance (RDA)
- Estimated Average Requirement (EAR)
- Adequate Intake (AI)

These recommendations create daily nutrient targets for building a healthy diet. I use these recommendations as a benchmark for determining the level of nutrients in foods and meals in this and the following section.

As explained in Section II, I do not agree with all the FNB's recommendations for **macronutrients**. Please know that the daily recommendations provided in this book that don't align with the FNB's are based on research from other highly credible health experts and organizations.

In Section III, I use all the FNB **micronutrient** daily recommendations as nutritional benchmarks, as these are accepted by nearly all credible nutrition information sources. There are no FNB recommendations for phytonutrients, as the science in this area is not sufficiently mature to make credible recommendations.

Macro and micronutrient measurement can be confusing. You should have a basic understanding of these measures so the book's dietary recommended strategies make sense.

The metric system is used to measure macro and micronutrients. The basic measure starts with grams. For background, 1 ounce is approximately 28 grams. Most macronutrients are measured in grams. Micronutrients are usually measured in milligrams (mg), equal to 1,000[th] of a gram, or micrograms (mcg), equal to 1 millionth of a gram. We're talking small amounts!

Lastly, I encourage you to read all five of the chapters in this section. I know this is a lot of information, but this is a great background to help you understand the nutritional value of common foods and make more informed food decisions. There is no test at the end, so there is no need to memorize all of this.

I think you might also be surprised to learn that many of the most nutritious foods are affordable and available at your local grocery stores. You are likely already consuming several of them.

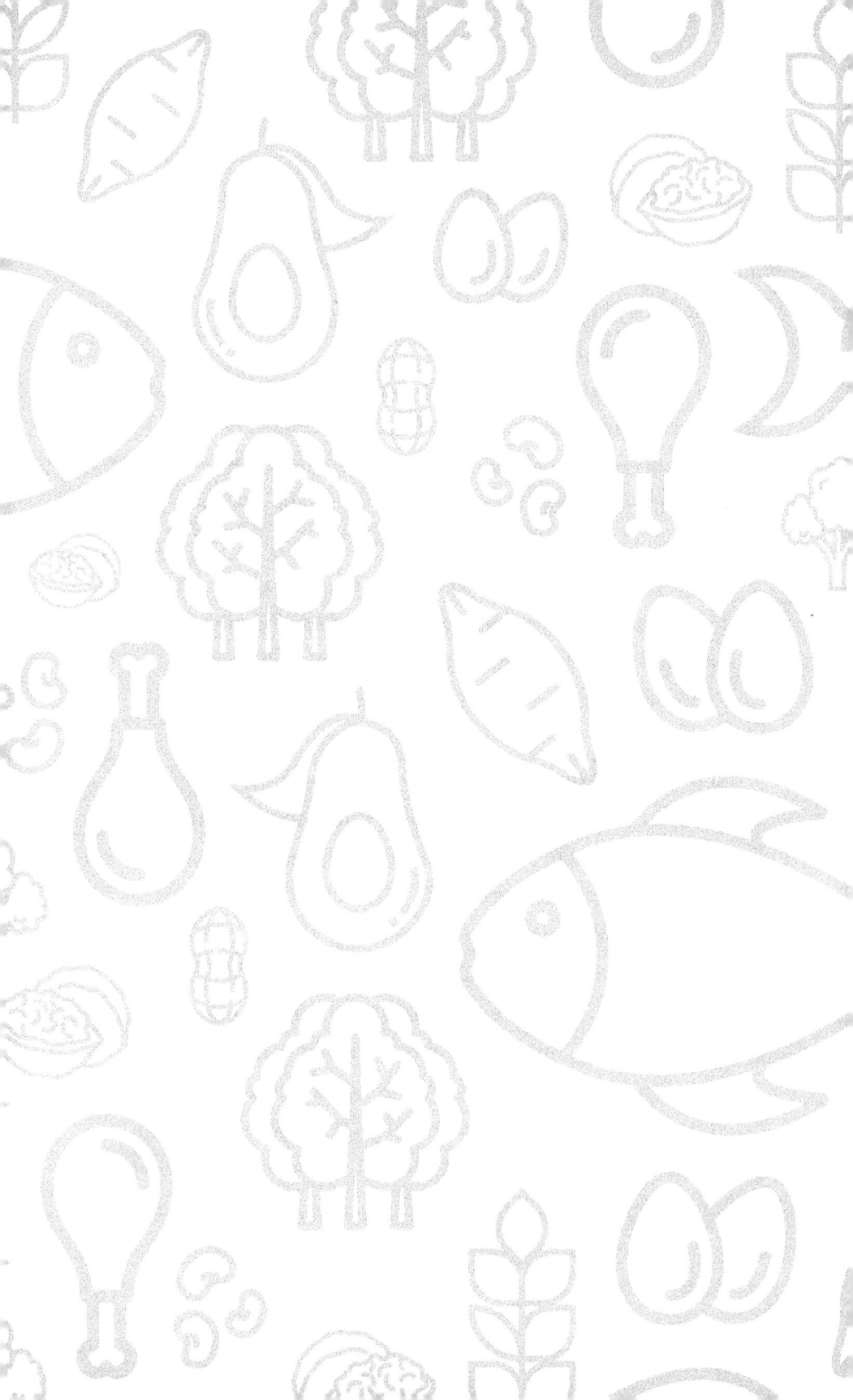

CHAPTER 12

Food Analyses and Organization

T o establish macronutrient benchmarks for measuring each food's nutrient levels, I used an average person's daily recommended caloric intake of 2,500 calories. This calorie count is based on national surveys that define the average American female and male in terms of height, weight, etc. I do this because a few of the book's macronutrient recommendations are based on a percentage of daily calories.

For micronutrients, I used the FNB's recommended DRIs as the benchmark. When there were different micronutrient recommendations for adult men versus adult women and the difference was minor, I averaged them. This was the case for all except iron. For iron, I used both the male and female recommendations as two separate benchmarks, as their difference was significant (18mg for women vs. 8mg for men).

For calculating all food nutrient levels, I used the USDA FoodData Central website and searched the "legacy foods" section. This is the website's section with the most comprehensive set of food nutrient analyses and is considered one of the most credible food nutrient databases in the world. To calculate accurate nutrient levels, I used the FoodData Central's nutrients per 100 grams for each food and adjusted for typical U.S. serving sizes.

I then compared each food's individual nutrient levels to the daily macro and micronutrient benchmarks described in previous sections. From this comparison, I calculated a nutrient level percentage. I categorized each food's individual nutrient levels into a scale. A food contains "very high" levels of a nutrient when it provides 50% or more of the daily recommendation, "high" levels when providing 20–49%, "moderate" at 10–29%, "low" at below 10%.

I know this sounds complicated, but I want you to have at least a basic understanding of my approach to these food analyses. Also, please understand that there are no perfectly nutritious foods. My goal was simply to identify those that are the *most* nutritious overall. The criteria I used to identify these nutrient-dense foods are:

- High levels of at least one macronutrient, prioritizing protein, unsaturated fats, and fiber.
- Unsaturated fat to saturated fat levels at a ratio of at least 2:1.
- Moderate to high levels of several vitamins, including choline.
- Moderate to high levels of several of the priority minerals: magnesium, potassium, iron, zinc, and calcium.

Many of the foods described in the next few chapters are not nutrient-dense but are still nutritious. I include these foods because a diet restricted to only nutrient-dense foods would be too limiting. There are simply not enough of them, and I don't believe most of us would stick to such a restrictive diet.

Food Breakdown

The next three chapters describe two types of food: animal-based and plant-based. Both types are important nutritionally and have different strengths and weaknesses.

I further break these into food groups, subsequently identifying the most nutritious foods within each group. For each one, I provide an overview of its nutrient content and my assessment of whether it's a nutrient-dense food that belongs on the last chapter's top 10 food list.

Because of the high volume of plant-based foods, I divided these into two chapters to make the information easier to get through.

All of the foods described in these chapters are supported by several credible nutritional and health sources. These include the U.S. Dietary Guidelines of Americans (DGA) report, the American Diabetes Association, American Heart Association, American Cancer Society, Centers for Disease Control and Prevention (CDC), leading U.S. medical schools, and several credible healthcare publications.

Additional sources used for food analyses description: [173] [174] [175]

CHAPTER 13

Animal-Based Foods

F ish, shellfish, chicken, eggs, dairy, and red meat are all animal-based foods. Most are highly nutritious, and several qualify as nutrient-dense. For good health, you should select animal foods that are either not processed or have low levels of processing. Examples of low-processed foods include cuts of meat in the butcher's section of your grocery store, packaged chicken cuts in the refrigerated section, and frozen whole shrimp.

If your food is pre-packaged or in a can, refer to the nutrition facts label to ensure you are not selecting a highly processed food. Those that are highly processed often contain a large number of ingredients, some of which you will not recognize (unless you are a chemist). Try to select options where the ingredients listed are almost exclusively natural and no or low in sodium, added sugar, artificial sweeteners, artificial coloring, and preservatives.

At typical serving sizes, unprocessed or low processed animal-based foods naturally have moderate to very high levels of protein, and low levels of carbohydrates, sugars, and sodium.

In terms of micronutrients, these animal foods usually contain high levels of several B vitamins and choline. A few have healthy levels of vitamins A and D. Animal foods are also typically moderate to high in the priority minerals magnesium, potassium, iron, and zinc.

While very nutritious, animal foods are typically low in a few important nutrients, notably fiber; vitamins B9 (folate), C, E, and K; and the minerals calcium and manganese. Other than a couple of animal food exceptions, you will need to get these nutrients from plant foods or supplements.

Saturated and Unsaturated Fat

Saturated and unsaturated fats are very important to good health. However, when saturated fat is consumed above recommended levels, certain health issues are a concern. Numerous studies show that diets high in saturated fat increase the risk of cardiovascular diseases. Such diets increase the chances of high blood pressure and atherosclerosis (plaque buildup in blood vessels). These health conditions are very common among many Americans and can shorten lifespan.

While there are a few contrary opinions on saturated fats, most credible nutritional experts, including the FNB and AHA, recommend limiting your daily intake. Many animal foods, especially red meat, tend to be high in saturated fats.

There is no debate on unsaturated fats, which are almost universally believed by experts to be very good for our health.

Studies have found that these fats support good cardiovascular, blood sugar, and brain health, among other things.

Most animal foods have moderate to high levels of monounsaturated fats. Fatty fish and seafood are high in polyunsaturated fats, in particular important omega-3 EPA/DHA. Eggs and some chicken cuts are good sources of the polyunsaturated fats omega-6 and omega-3 ALA. Many red meats and dairy are low in polyunsaturated fats.

Based on FNB recommendations for dietary fats overall, a healthy diet should include twice as much unsaturated fat as saturated fat. Unfortunately, some animal foods do not reach this 2:1 ratio and can pose health risks if consumed regularly.

Does this mean that you should not eat animal-based foods? Absolutely not. These foods are very nutritious and part of a balanced diet. Also, there are several animal foods with a good to very good fat profiles above the 2:1 ratio; many of these are on my list of the most nutrient-dense foods. However, you need to moderate your intake of animal foods that are high in saturated fat.

Now, let's look at the healthiest animal foods.

Fatty Fish

Fresh fatty fish, like salmon, tuna, rainbow trout, and sardines, are nutrient-dense. A 6-ounce serving of these fish has approximately 200–350 calories and includes high levels of protein (>20%, <50% of DRI) at 40–50 grams per serving. They are low in carbohydrates (<10% of DRI), natural sugar, sodium, and fiber.

These fish also have some of the healthiest animal food fat profiles. While they have moderate levels of saturated fats (>10%, <20% of DRI), they are uniquely very high in important omega-3 EPA and DHA (>50% of DRI), and moderate to high in healthy monounsaturated fats. Some also have moderate to high levels of omega-3 ALA.

Most fatty fish have 2–2.5 times the amount of unsaturated fats compared to saturated fats, which is very good. Sardines and salmon have even healthier fat profiles, better than many plant foods.

The vitamin profile of these fatty fish is also outstanding, featuring very high levels of vitamin D and moderate to high levels of vitamins A and E, several B vitamins, and choline. The vitamin D levels should be highlighted, as fatty fish are one of the few food sources for this critical vitamin.

As for minerals, fatty fish have moderate to high levels of magnesium, potassium, zinc, and iron. Tuna and sardines provide high amounts of iron for men and moderate amounts for women. Tuna also has moderate levels of iodine, while some canned versions of salmon and sardines contain high levels of calcium.

All of these fish are nutrient-dense, but if I had to pick the best it would be salmon. Its combination of high protein, a great fat profile, and being full of many vitamins and minerals make it a great food option to regularly include in your diet. Salmon is highlighted in my list of **top 10 foods** in the last chapter of this section.

Sardines, tuna, and rainbow trout are also very nutritious. These make my **honorable mention** list in the last chapter.

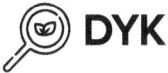

DYK

Tilapia is cheaper and nutritionally similar to fatty fish. It has moderate to high levels of magnesium, potassium, selenium, most B vitamins, choline, and vitamin D, but is low in healthy unsaturated fats. There are some health concerns with farmed tilapia. If not wild caught, buy farmed tilapia from the U.S., Canada, the Netherlands, Ecuador, or Peru as the countries of origin.

Lastly, try to avoid or limit fish known to be high in mercury. These include shark, swordfish, king mackerel, marlin, big-eyed tuna, orange roughy, and tilefish (Gulf of Mexico). Focus instead on consuming fish with lower levels, such as salmon, canned light tuna, sardines, tilapia, pollock, and catfish.

📖 Highly Processed Foods Facts Break

I analyzed the nutrient value of a fast-food fish sandwich with tartar sauce and cheese. I compared it to a sandwich made of 3 ounces of canned pink salmon with hummus, chopped red sweet peppers, and chopped celery on two slices of 100% whole-wheat bread. Here's what I found:

- → *The fried fish sandwich costs approximately $5. The salmon sandwich totaled $6.50. I bought this canned wild salmon in bulk online with no added salt.*

- → *The fried fish sandwich had moderate levels of protein and had a very good fat profile with 3 times unsaturated fats to saturated fats. It also had high levels of a few B vitamins and moderate levels of vitamin K and the minerals magnesium, potassium, iron, and calcium.*

- → *However, the salmon sandwich had over 2 times the protein, 8 times the fiber, 2 times or more the levels of most B vitamins, 3 times the vitamin K, 4 times the vitamins A and E, 10 times the vitamin D, and 50 times the vitamin C. It also had over 2 times or more magnesium, potassium, iron, and calcium. Its fat profile was also better.*

- → *In addition to being much less nutritious, the fried sandwich had close to 2 times more sodium and saturated fat than the salmon sandwich.*

Shellfish

Shellfish include clams, crab, crayfish, lobster, mussels, oysters, scallops, shrimp, and squid. They are a nutritious food group, but not as nutrient-dense as fatty fish.

Oysters, clams, and shrimp are three of the most nutritious examples of shellfish. Typical sizes vary based on the shellfish.

Shellfish are low in calories, provide moderate levels of protein, and are low in saturated fat. They also have moderate levels of important omega-3 EPA/DHA. Their fat profile is not as good as fatty fish, as they are much lower in unsaturated fats overall.

Their vitamin profile includes moderate to high levels of several B vitamins and very high levels of B12. Most shellfish are also moderate in vitamin E and high in choline.

As for minerals, as a group they have moderate to high amounts of zinc, with oysters being extremely high (<100% of DRI). Oysters and claims both have high levels of iron, with high amounts for men and moderate to high levels for women. Clams are uniquely high in potassium and vitamins A and C.

One drawback is that clams and shrimp are naturally high in sodium, so they are best consumed in moderate portions.

Unless you are allergic to these foods, shellfish are a healthy addition to your diet. The U.S. government recommends adults consume two servings of seafood (fish and shellfish) per week. Most shellfish have low levels of mercury.

Fresh Poultry

Poultry includes chicken and turkey, which have very similar nutritional profiles. Chicken is now the most consumed meat in the U.S.

Poultry is very nutritious and moderate in calories at 250–350 per 6-ounce serving. In terms of its macronutrient profile, it is high in protein with 40–50 grams and low in carbohydrates, natural sugar, and fiber.

Most poultry cuts have moderate to high levels of saturated fat and moderate to high levels of monounsaturated fats, omega-6, and omega-3 ALA. This translates to a good fat profile with approximately twice as many unsaturated fats as saturated fats.

Poultry has high to very high levels of several B vitamins and choline. It has moderate levels of vitamin K2. It also has moderate to high amounts of magnesium, potassium, zinc, and iron. Like many animal foods, it is high in phosphorus and selenium.

Healthy cuts of chicken include the breasts, legs, and thighs. Chicken breast is highest in protein and lowest in saturated fat. Chicken thighs and legs have many of the same nutrients as chicken breasts, but are higher in saturated fat, monounsaturated fats, omega-6, and zinc. With higher saturated and unsaturated fat levels, thighs and legs still have a good fat profile, slightly better than breasts.

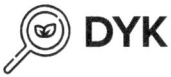

⊙ DYK

Duck and goose generally have as high or even higher levels of nutrients than chicken and turkey. Unfortunately, they also are much higher in saturated fat and calories. If you enjoy these foods, make them an occasional treat and exercise portion control.

With its high levels of nutrients, healthy fat profile, and lower cost relative to other meats, chicken should be part of your regular diet. It's one of my top 10 list of most nutritious foods.

Eggs

Chicken eggs are very nutritious. A two-egg serving has only 150 calories and is a moderate source of protein. A three-egg serving has protein levels close to high.

Eggs do have moderate levels of saturated fat but twice the levels of unsaturated fats, which makes for a good fat profile. Despite their reputation, eggs have not been found to cause high blood cholesterol in healthy individuals.

Eggs contain several vitamins, including moderate to high levels of several B vitamins. They are one of the few animal foods that contain moderate levels of B9. In addition, eggs have high levels of vitamin A and moderate levels of vitamins D and E (assuming a serving size of three eggs). They include very high levels of the important nutrient choline.

As for minerals, a two-egg serving has high levels of iron for men (moderate for women) and moderate levels of zinc. Lastly, they contain the phytonutrient carotenoids lutein and zeaxanthin.

If you are currently not eating eggs, I recommend you add them as a part of your regular diet. They are high in many nutrients that Americans struggle to get at adequate levels. When you factor in their lower cost relative to other animal food options, they are a great choice. They are on my top 10 list of the most nutritious foods.

🏅 Pro Move

The protein in cooked eggs is 180% more digestible than raw eggs. Cook those eggies![176]

Dairy

Dairy comes in a variety of products, including milk, yogurt, cheese, kefir, ice cream, butter, cottage cheese, cream, sour cream, cream cheese, whey protein powder, etc. It is a good source of a few important nutrients but doesn't qualify as nutrient dense.

Some of the healthiest dairy products are plain Greek yogurt, plain kefir, unflavored milk, and cottage cheese. A typical serving of these products is 100–150 calories (less for kefir) and is low to moderate in protein. Greek yogurt and cottage cheese provide the highest amounts of protein, reaching moderate to high levels.

Full-fat dairy products are moderate to high in saturated fat. They are also low in monounsaturated fat and omega-6, and have moderate amounts of omega-3 ALA. They have a poor fat profile with half the levels of unsaturated fats compared to saturated fats, or a .5:1 ratio.

Low-fat and no-fat dairy products have slightly higher protein levels and about the same levels of vitamins and minerals. Many health and nutrition experts recommend moving to low- and no-fat dairy products for adults to reduce saturated fat intake, but this may not be warranted. When dairy fat is lowered, both saturated and unsaturated fat levels are decreased, which translates to the approximately the same poor fat ratio.

The good news is that several credible health sources state that two to three daily servings of full fat dairy a day are healthy. These studies show that the saturated fat in dairy does not have the same negative health impact as other high saturated fat foods with poor fat ratios. In these studies, dairy was *not* associated with poor cardiovascular health, type 2 diabetes, or weight gain.[177] [178]

In terms of vitamin profile, dairy has high levels of B2 and B12 and moderate amounts of B5. Unless fortified, it has low levels of all other vitamins, except for kefir, which is high in vitamin A. Milk is often fortified with vitamins A and D. Also, some hard cheeses are moderate to high in K2.

As for minerals, dairy deserves its reputation of providing calcium, as it has moderate to high levels, depending on the product. It is one of the very few food sources for this important mineral. Dairy also has low to moderate levels of zinc.

Note that plain Greek yogurt and kefir are fermented and provide high levels of probiotics. These support a healthy gut microbiota. Studies show that these dairy products reduce atherosclerosis (buildup of plaque in arteries) which is one of the greatest risks of high saturated fat consumption. Of all dairy selections, these may be the best to regularly consume.

🏅 Pro Move

If your budget allows, try grass-fed dairy products. Studies show these are higher than regular dairy in omega-3 ALA and omega-6 fatty acids as well as vitamins A and E. This advice also applies to other animal foods as well.

Lastly, whey protein powder is another dairy-based product. It has become very popular over the last few decades for active people and athletes to increase their daily protein intake. There are approximately 25–40 grams of protein per serving, depending on the whey protein product. It is typically low in saturated fat, added sugar, and calories, but make sure to review the nutrition facts label to verify this.

The advantage of whey protein powder is that it is easily added to yogurt, oatmeal, smoothies, etc. If you are struggling to achieve your daily recommended protein levels, consider adding whey protein to your diet.

If you are a vegetarian, pea protein powder is a good alternative.

Fresh Red Meat

Red meat includes beef, pork, lamb, bison, and wild game. Fresh red meat is not processed or has low processing. It is nutrient-dense but has one significant nutritional flaw in that most cuts of red meat have high to very high levels of saturated fat.

Further, red meat has a poor to very poor fat profile, depending on the type of animal and cut. Even lean cuts have unsaturated fat levels approximately the same as their saturated fat levels. This translates to a poor fat ratio of close to 1:1. The exception is lean pork chops, with a ratio of more than 2:1.

Red meat is a great source of protein. At a 6-ounce serving size, it also has high to very high levels of most B vitamins (not B9 folate) and choline. It contains moderate to high levels of the minerals magnesium, potassium, iron (men and women), and zinc.

Given the diseases linked to high intake of red meat and saturated fat in several studies, it is difficult to recommend red meat as a frequent food source.[179] [180] [181] If you regularly consume highly processed red meat foods (think sausage, bacon, etc.) the risk of disease is even greater. These foods are associated with early mortality, cancer, and diabetes.

Some recent studies show that limited intake (two servings per week) of unprocessed, fresh red meat is not associated with some of these health risks. Unfortunately, most credible health-care sources do not agree with these studies at this time.

So, does this mean I recommend not eating red meat? For many in the U.S., red meat is one of their top dinner entrees and consumed regularly. It would be tough for them to go completely "cold turkey" on red meat (although cold turkey does have a much better fat profile!).

It is really an individual decision, but I don't think you need to eliminate fresh red meat from your diet entirely. However, if you are going to eat red meat with any regularity, I recommend you consider the following strategies to reduce health risks:

- **Select lean, unprocessed cuts at moderate portion sizes**. The red meat options described below are all lean cuts. They have lower levels of calories and saturated fats than most other cuts.
- **Limit red meat to no more than one serving a week.** This may be difficult at first, but there are a lot of other nutritious, delicious animal foods recommended above to fill out your diet. Make red meat an occasional treat.
- **Try trimming off the fat.** Eliminating extra fat on the outside of the meat significantly lowers levels of saturated fat.
- **Give game meats a try.** Wild game meats typically have a better fat profile than other red meats and are higher in iron and omega-3 ALA.

- **Add foods to your diet with great fat profiles.**
  Foods like avocados, peanuts, soybeans, nuts, and olive
  oil will help you balance out your overall diet's fat profile
  and support better health. These all have 4x or more the
  levels of unsaturated fat compared to saturated fat.

Below is a list of some of the healthiest cuts from a saturated
fat perspective. These descriptions are based on a moderate
6-ounce serving size:

Beef: Healthier cuts of beef include top sirloin, flank steak,
and many of the "round" cuts. Also, filet mignon is a relatively
healthy cut of beef. These meats have approximately 300–350
calories, 45–50 grams of protein, and moderate saturated fat
levels, and are particularly high in B6 and B12.

Except for filet mignon, these cuts can be tougher than
higher fat options, so try marinating them and/or slow cooking
to tenderize the meat. There are lots of great recipes on
the internet.

As for ground beef, try to select options with 10% fat or less.
This places the saturated fat at healthier levels.

Pork: Pork tenderloin and center cut pork chops are healthier
choices. A serving size has approximately 250–350 calories and
45 grams of protein, and is particularly high in vitamins B1, B2,
B5, and B6. A lean pork tenderloin is low in saturated fat.

Lamb: Many cuts of lamb are high in saturated fat, but lamb tenderloin and trimmed hind shank are at healthier levels. Per serving, lamb has approximately 300–350 calories and 50 grams of protein, provides over 100% of the daily recommendation of B12, and has moderate amounts of omega-3 ALA.

Wild game: Deer, elk, and bison all have a nutritional profile similar to beef. Their wild existence and natural diet make them unique in that they tend to be slightly lower in calories and saturated fat, and higher in iron. Wild game also has slightly higher polyunsaturated fat omega-3 ALA.

Organ meat: If you can stomach it (pun intended), consider adding organ meat to your diet occasionally. These meats include liver, tongue, and heart. They are some of the most nutrient-dense protein foods on the planet and have very high levels (over 100%) of many important minerals and vitamin A.

Note that if you are pregnant or have high cholesterol or gout, you should consult with your doctor before adding organ meats to your regular diet.

My Animal-Based Foods Approach

I consume a variety of animal-based foods weekly and focus on those most nutrient-dense with good fat profiles. I eat these foods mostly at dinner, with some dairy at breakfast (Greek yogurt and kefir) for calcium and to support gut health.

For my dinners, I have fatty fish approximately twice per week, poultry two to three times (both breast and thighs), three eggs one to two times per week, and lean ground beef or bison once a week. My serving sizes for meat are typically 6–8 ounces. I avoid food monotony by making different types of dishes with these meats, regularly preparing the meals described in the last section of this book.

These animal-based food selections help me meet the daily recommendations for protein, unsaturated fats (particularly hard to get omega-3 EPA/DHA), B vitamins, vitamins A and D, choline, and several priority minerals. To attain the remaining important nutrient DRIs, I rely on plant foods.

📖 Highly Processed Foods Facts Break

I analyzed a fast-food cheeseburger's nutrients. Here's what I found:

→ *The beef and cheese provide moderate levels of protein and unsaturated fats and high levels of vitamins B1, B2, B3, B12, and choline. It has healthy levels of iron, zinc, and calcium.*

→ *Unfortunately, like most fast foods, it is very high in sodium and saturated fats.*

→ *Let's say you added a regular order of fries and 12-ounce cola to this meal and then had one more cheeseburger and a drink refill (not uncommon for fast food). This meal would then provide over the recommended daily sodium limit by 25%, 2.5 times the daily added sugar limit, and 75% of the daily saturated fat limit. This one meal would also have a total of over 1,400 calories!*

→ *A meal such as this does have some nutrients, but it exposes you to dangerously high levels of others.*

→ *It is also low in most vitamins and fiber. This meal falls far short of nutrient-dense and will make it difficult to reach the DRI of several important nutrients the day consumed.*

Additional sources used for animal foods description: [182] [183] [184] [185] [186] [187] [188] [189]

CHAPTER 14

Vegetables and Fruits

P lant-based whole foods include vegetables, fruits, legumes, nuts, and seeds. By whole foods, I mean they have no or minimal processing and are free or nearly free of additives.

In typical serving sizes, plant foods are great sources of complex carbohydrates and fiber, and low to moderate in natural sugar. Almost all plant foods have a healthy fat profile, as they are typically low in saturated fat, and several contain healthy amounts of unsaturated fats. Plant foods generally are low in calories, protein, and sodium.

In addition, they are an important source of vitamins A, B9, C, E, and K, as well as most priority minerals. Plant-based foods are also the best sources of phytonutrients and their antioxidants.

If your diet is exclusively comprised of plant foods, you will find it challenging to get adequate levels of omega-3 EPA/DHA, vitamin B12, vitamin D, and choline. Additionally, few plant foods have healthy levels of calcium and selenium.

You will also need to be intentional in your diet about getting up to my recommended levels of daily protein. You may consider using plant-based protein powder or other high protein processed plant-based products to boost your levels. Please always look at the nutrient facts labels on these products to ensure they do not contain unhealthy levels of additives.

Many of the plant-based foods described in this section are nutrient-dense and a key part of a healthy diet.

Vegetables

Vegetables are a versatile food group and can be prepared raw, stir-fried, roasted, or steamed. They are a great source of complex carbohydrates, several vitamins, fiber, phytonutrients, and antioxidants. They are typically low in calories, protein, saturated fats, and unsaturated fats.

DYK

Whole vegetables are the edible parts of plants such as their leaves, stems, roots, and bulbs. There are more than 1,000 varieties of vegetables.

Below is a list of some of the healthiest and most consumed vegetables in the U.S.

Cruciferous Vegetables

Broccoli, kale, and brussels sprouts all belong to this plant family, along with cabbage and cauliflower. This group is also referred to as brassica. Broccoli, brussels sprouts, and kale have the most significant amounts of nutrients in this food group.

A single serving size of 1 cup of cooked broccoli, kale, or brussels sprouts ($\frac{1}{2}$ cup) provides low levels of calories, protein, natural sugars, and fats. Broccoli and kale also provide moderate amounts of omega-3 ALA. They all provide moderate amounts of fiber.

Cruciferous vegetables stand out nutritionally with their vitamin, phytonutrient, and antioxidant levels. They have high to very high levels of vitamins C and K, and moderate to high amounts of vitamins A, B2, B6, and B9. They also contain the phytonutrients organosulfur compounds, carotenoids, and phenolic acids.

While these vegetables are similar, they do have slightly different nutritional profiles. Cooked kale is especially high in vitamins A and K. Cooked broccoli is higher in B5 and B6. Both provide moderate amounts of vitamin E.

As for minerals, the group provides moderate amounts of iron (men only), magnesium, and potassium. Kale also has high levels of calcium.

Cooked broccoli and kale (and their raw versions) are nutrient-dense and the most nutritious cruciferous vegetables. Both are on my list of top 10 foods.

Leafy Greens

Leafy greens are great for making salads, sandwiches, or adding to soups. Though not nutrient-dense, they are a great nutritional complement when added to meals. Overall, leafy greens are very low in calories, protein, carbohydrates, fats, and fiber.

As a group, a one-cup raw serving size provides a few important vitamins and minerals. Some of the most nutritious leafy greens are spinach, romaine, green and butter/bibb lettuce, and swiss chard. These greens have high to very high levels of vitamin K and moderate to high levels of vitamins B9 and A.

They are low to moderate in iron (men only).

Cooked spinach is the most nutritious of the group. A ⅓-cup serving (cooked down from two cups raw) has the nutrients listed above, plus moderate levels of vitamins B2 and B6. It also has high levels of iron (moderate for women) and moderate levels of magnesium and potassium.

In addition, spinach contains the phytonutrients flavonoids, carotenoids, and phenolic acid. This pushes it close to nutrient-dense territory.

Overall, leafy greens are a healthy addition to any meal.

In case you are wondering, iceberg lettuce is very low in almost all nutrients. It does have moderate amounts of vitamin K.

Asparagus

This is another nutritious green vegetable. A ½-cup serving (three to four spears) cooked is low in calories, protein, fiber, natural sugar, and all fats.

Its nutritional value comes from its high levels of vitamin K and B9. It also has moderate amounts of vitamins B1, B2, C, and E. In addition, asparagus has moderate levels of iron (men only), copper, and selenium.

Asparagus also contains the phytonutrients beta-carotene, lutein, and zeaxanthin. While not a nutrient-dense food, asparagus is a nutritious food.

Root Vegetables

These vegetables are nutritious, but some are significantly higher in nutrients than others. With their differing nutritional profiles, it's best to eat a variety to get the most complete benefit. Below is a summary of each root vegetable's nutrients:

Sweet potatoes are delicious, easy to prepare, and very healthy. They are a nutrient-dense food.

Try eating them with their skins, as this adds to their levels of nutrients and fiber. One medium baked sweet potato is low in calories, protein, and carbohydrates, and has moderate levels of fiber and natural sugar.

In terms of vitamins, a sweet potato (with skin) is very high in vitamin A (>100% of DRI). It also provides high levels of vitamins C, B5, and B6 and moderate levels of B1, B2, and B3.

This vegetable further contains moderate levels of magnesium, potassium, and iron (men only). Lastly, it's the highest vegetable in the phytonutrient beta-carotene and contains the phytonutrient resveratrol.

With all these nutrients, sweet potatoes should be a regular addition to your diet. They are on my top 10 list of most nutritious foods.

Potatoes are another healthy root vegetable. A medium-sized potato with the skin is low in calories and protein. It is moderate in carbohydrates and fiber, and has high levels of vitamins C and B6 and moderate amounts of several other B vitamins.

As for minerals, a potato has high levels of iron (moderate for women), potassium, and copper. It has moderate amounts of magnesium and manganese.

Potatoes are also high in starch, with over twice the level of sweet potatoes. These are nutritious vegetables but are not quite nutrient dense.

⊚ Pro Move

Many starchy foods (potatoes, whole wheat pasta, etc.) are high in what is called resistant starch. Cooking breaks down these starches into simple sugars, which are then absorbed quickly by the body. This can cause high blood sugar. Studies show that when cooled overnight and reheated, much of the resistant starch returns, reducing simple sugars. This reduces glucose absorption significantly, lowering the associated health risk.

Carrots, raw or cooked, have very similar nutrients. A serving size of ⅔ cup is very low in calories, protein, and carbohydrates. It is high in vitamin A and the phytonutrient beta-carotene. In addition, carrots have moderate amounts of vitamins K and B6 and, when raw, the mineral potassium.

Carrots are not as high in natural sugar as is commonly thought. They contain approximately 3–5 grams per serving, which is low, and given their fiber content should not be a health concern. Overall, carrots are a healthy addition to your diet.

Beets are high in B9 and low in other vitamins. They are also moderate in iron (men only), potassium, and manganese. Beets contain nitrate compounds that may be helpful in lowering blood pressure. Beets are moderate in natural sugar. A serving size is considered to be ¾ cup.

Onions are delicious in a variety of dishes and are also nutritious. They are low in protein, carbohydrates, natural sugar, and fiber, but contain types of soluble fiber that are a good prebiotic for our gut microbiota. A serving size of onions (½ cup) contains moderate levels of vitamins B6 and C (raw only). Onions also contain phytonutrient flavonoids.

Lastly, onions (and garlic, shallots, leeks, and chives) contain allyl sulfides. These phytonutrients are believed to have many potential health benefits.

Fermented vegetables should also be considered for your diet. In addition to providing the vegetable nutrients, these are excellent probiotics for gut health. Examples of these foods are pickled sauerkraut from cabbage, and pickled cucumbers, carrots, and cauliflower.

📖 Vegetables Facts Break

Many of the vegetables we consume today have been culti-vated for thousands of years.

→ *Cruciferous vegetables were first grown in ancient Greece and Rome.*

→ *Potatoes and sweet potatoes (and tomatoes) orig-inated from South America over 4,000 years ago.*

→ *Spinach is believed to be first cultivated in Persia over 2,000 years ago.*

→ *Carrots are believed to originate from the Middle East over 5,000 years ago.*

→ *Ancient literature from China, India, Greece, and Egypt cite the medicinal and therapeutic applica-tions of garlic and onions.*

→ *The practice of fermenting vegetables as a means of preservation is believed to date back some 10,000 years.*

Fruits

Whole fruits are nutritious, delicious, and a great source of complex carbohydrates. Like vegetables, fruits have a wide variety of nutritional profiles.

Fruits often have the reputation for being high in natural sugar and they are relative to most other food groups. However, at normal serving sizes, very few provide levels that should be a concern for high blood sugar. When consumed in their natural state, most have healthy amounts of fiber to help slow the sugar's absorption into the bloodstream.

In fact, several studies show that regular consumption of fruits supports healthy blood sugar levels and weight management. If you do have diabetes or prediabetes, consult your physician on dietary strategies including fruit consumption.

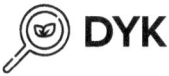

DYK

Whole fruits are typically from the flowering part of a plant or tree and are sweet, fleshy, and seed bearing. There are over 2,000 varieties of fruits worldwide.

Below is a list of some of the most nutritious fruits commonly consumed in the U.S.

Avocados

Avocados check a lot of nutritional boxes. One medium avocado is relatively high in calories, at approximately 240. It is low in protein, carbohydrates, and natural sugar. It contains high levels of fiber.

Avocados are a unique fruit due to their fat profile. They contain moderate amounts of saturated fat, but also have very high amounts of monounsaturated fats as well as moderate amounts of omega-6 and omega-3 ALA fats. The result is an excellent fat profile with over 5 times the amount of unsaturated fats compared to saturated fat.

Avocados also have a very good vitamin profile with high levels of B5, B6, B9, E, and K. In addition, they have moderate amounts of vitamins B1, B2, B3, and C. Avocados are high in potassium, and have moderate levels of magnesium, zinc, and iron (men only).

Avocados are a nutritional powerhouse, and if you are not eating them already, you should start. They are on my top 10 list of the most nutritious foods.

Berries

Blueberries, strawberries, blackberries, raspberries, and kiwis all have healthy nutritional profiles. A 1-cup serving (or 1 medium kiwi) has low levels of calories, protein, carbs, and most fats. These fruits contain moderate to high amounts of fiber and are low to moderate in omega-3 ALA.

They also provide several additional important nutrients, but these vary significantly by berry. In terms of vitamins, they have moderate to high levels of vitamins C (with strawberries and kiwi containing the highest levels), K (highest in kiwi and blueberries) and B9 (strawberries and blackberries having the highest levels).

Strawberries, blackberries, and raspberries contain moderate amounts of iron (men only).

Berries are considered very high in antioxidants, with several different types of flavonoids. They also contain phenolic acids and the phytoestrogen resveratrol.

Berries don't have the macronutrient and micronutrient profiles to be a considered a top nutrient-dense food, but their phytonutrient content pushes them into nutrient-dense territory. Accordingly, I have placed them on my list of honorable mentions for nutrient-dense foods.

Note that grapes are also considered a berry, but their macro and micronutrient profiles fall slightly below these others. They are high in phytonutrients and are a healthy addition to your diet. However, they are much higher in sugar than other berries.

Citrus Fruits

Oranges, lemons, grapefruits, and tangerines are the most consumed citrus fruits in the U.S. They are low in calories, protein, carbs, and all fats. A few have moderate levels of fiber. I do not consider them a nutrient-dense food because of their overall low vitamin and mineral levels.

At typical serving sizes, citrus fruits are nutritionally important because of their very high levels of vitamin C. As previously discussed, this water-soluble vitamin is needed daily. It is also a strong antioxidant.

Citrus fruits' nutritional values vary by fruit. Per serving, oranges have the highest levels of vitamin C (100% of the DRI) and are moderate in fiber, B1, B9, and potassium. Tangerines have a similar nutritional profile.

Grapefruits are also very high in vitamin C and moderate in vitamin A. Lemons are high in vitamin C and have low levels of all other micronutrients.

Citrus fruits contain several phytonutrients, including flavonoids. They also contain carotenoids and phenolic acids, with higher concentrations in their peels.

Several studies show that the vitamin C and phytonutrients in citrus may lower the risks of certain cancers, DNA damage, cardiovascular disease, diabetes, and inflammation.

Add citrus fruits to your diet. They are great to eat as a snack (just peel and eat), to add some pizazz to water, or to enhance certain meals. If you are not a citrus fruit fan, try pineapple instead. It has citrus-like nutritional properties and is very high in vitamin C.

🏅 Pro Move

If you want to increase your daily vitamin C, fiber, and phytonutrient levels, consider using the zest of your citrus peels in your morning water, afternoon smoothie, etc. These peels have significantly higher levels of vitamin C and phytonutrients per gram than the juice.

Peppers

Some of the most nutritious peppers are bell, sweet red, and red-hot chili. This is not a nutrient-dense food, but it is nutritious.

A serving of ⅔ cup of peppers is very low in calories, protein, all fats, and fiber. Their nutritional value is mostly in their vitamin C levels. One serving has well over 100% of the DRI.

In addition, peppers have moderate to high amounts of vitamins B6, B9, A, and E. Peppers are low in all essential minerals.

Peppers also contain the phytonutrients beta-carotene, lutein, and zeaxanthin; green peppers additionally contain the phytoestrogen lignans.

These fruits are easy to add into a salad, smoothie, chili, or stir fry. Please add them to your diet.

Tomatoes

Like many of the fruits described above, tomatoes are low in calories, protein, all fats, and fiber. Most tomato products have moderate to high levels of vitamin C and potassium. Their fat profile is very good, but they are low in unsaturated fats.

The nutrient density of tomato products increases when they are cooked, especially in pasta sauce and stewed tomatoes. A typical ½ cup of canned stewed tomatoes (for chili or soup) has moderate levels of vitamin C and potassium, and high levels of iron (moderate for women).

A full cup of tomato-based pasta sauce is very nutritious and has the same nutrients as stewed tomatoes, except at higher levels because of the higher quantity. It also contains moderate to high levels of vitamins B2, B3, B5, B6, and E, as well as the mineral magnesium.

In addition, tomatoes are the best food source of an important phytonutrient carotenoid called lycopene. An anti-oxidant, lycopene is believed to protect against certain cancers and other health risks.

Note that a full cup of healthy pasta sauce, even without high levels of additives, may be as high as 200 calories. Please factor this into your serving size decision. Your selection of pasta sauce is an important one. Many are high in added sodium and sugar. Refer to the nutrient facts label to select a sauce with low to moderate levels of added sugar and sodium.

Tomatoes are nearly at the nutrient-dense level but fall just short. They are a very nutritious food that you should have in your diet.

Stone Fruits

Cherries, peaches, and plums are some of the most consumed stone fruits in the U.S. These contain only a few important nutrients at healthy levels and therefore are not nutrient-dense.

A regular serving size would be 1 medium peach, 1½ plums, or ½ cup of pitted cherries. Per serving, these fruits have low to moderate amounts of vitamin C, potassium, and copper. They also contain phytonutrient carotenoids and flavonoids. They have moderate levels of natural sugar.

These foods are a healthy snack. Apricots and nectarines also fit into this fruit group and are similar nutritionally. Apricots are particularly high in vitamin A.

Bananas

Bananas are one of the most consumed fruits in the U.S. They are primarily known for their potassium levels but also contain healthy amounts of other important nutrients. They are low in protein and all fats and have moderate amounts of natural sugar.

One medium banana has high levels of vitamin B6 and moderate amounts of vitamin C, potassium, and manganese. It also has healthy soluble fiber.

They are not a nutrient-dense food but are a healthy fruit for your diet.

Apples

Apples are delicious and moderate in fiber, containing both soluble and insoluble fiber. They are low in macro and micro-nutrients but have several phytonutrient flavonoids. They are a healthy snack, but not nutrient-dense.

This is not an exhaustive list of nutritious fruits. Other healthy choices include mangos and pomegranates.

Fresh vs. Frozen vs. Canned vs. Dried Plant-Based Foods Facts Break

What's best for plant-based food for nutrition: fresh, frozen, or canned?

→ *Plant foods are most nutritious at harvest, but for most of us this isn't an option.*

→ *Fresh fruits and vegetables' nutrients degrade during transport to the grocery store. It varies by plant, but on average they lose 50% of their nutritional value. They also do degrade once in the refrigerator, but the cooler temperature slows this degrading.*

→ *Frozen fruits and vegetables are flash frozen within hours of harvesting. Vegetables are blanched before freezing, causing some nutrient loss. Once frozen, both retain most nutrients.*

→ *Canned fruits and vegetables are exposed to intense heat to kill microorganisms, which decreases nutrients, particularly water-soluble vitamins (C and Bs). Once in the can, they retain the remaining nutrients for long periods. Watch out for added sodium and sugar in canned foods.*

So, what's the best method nutritionally? More science is needed, but the following seems to be the consensus:

→ *Fresh is best for vitamin C-rich foods, such as citrus and peppers. Also, apples and pears.*

→ *Frozen seems to be best for vegetables, which maintain most nutrients.*

→ *Canned works well for carrots, pumpkin, and tomato products because these maintain most of their nutrients during heating. Some phytonutrients are even enhanced.*

→ *Nuts and seeds are dried or dry roasted after harvest and retain most nutrients for months.*

→ *Legumes are typically dried or canned and retain most of their nutrients for months.*

→ *Grains are dried after harvesting. If stored properly, they maintain most nutrients for several months.*

→ *For the best nutrient retention, nuts, seeds, legumes, and grains should all be stored in cool, dry places and in airtight containers once their package is opened.*

Additional sources used for vegetables and fruits description: [190] [191] [192] [193] [194] [195] [196] [197] [198] [199]

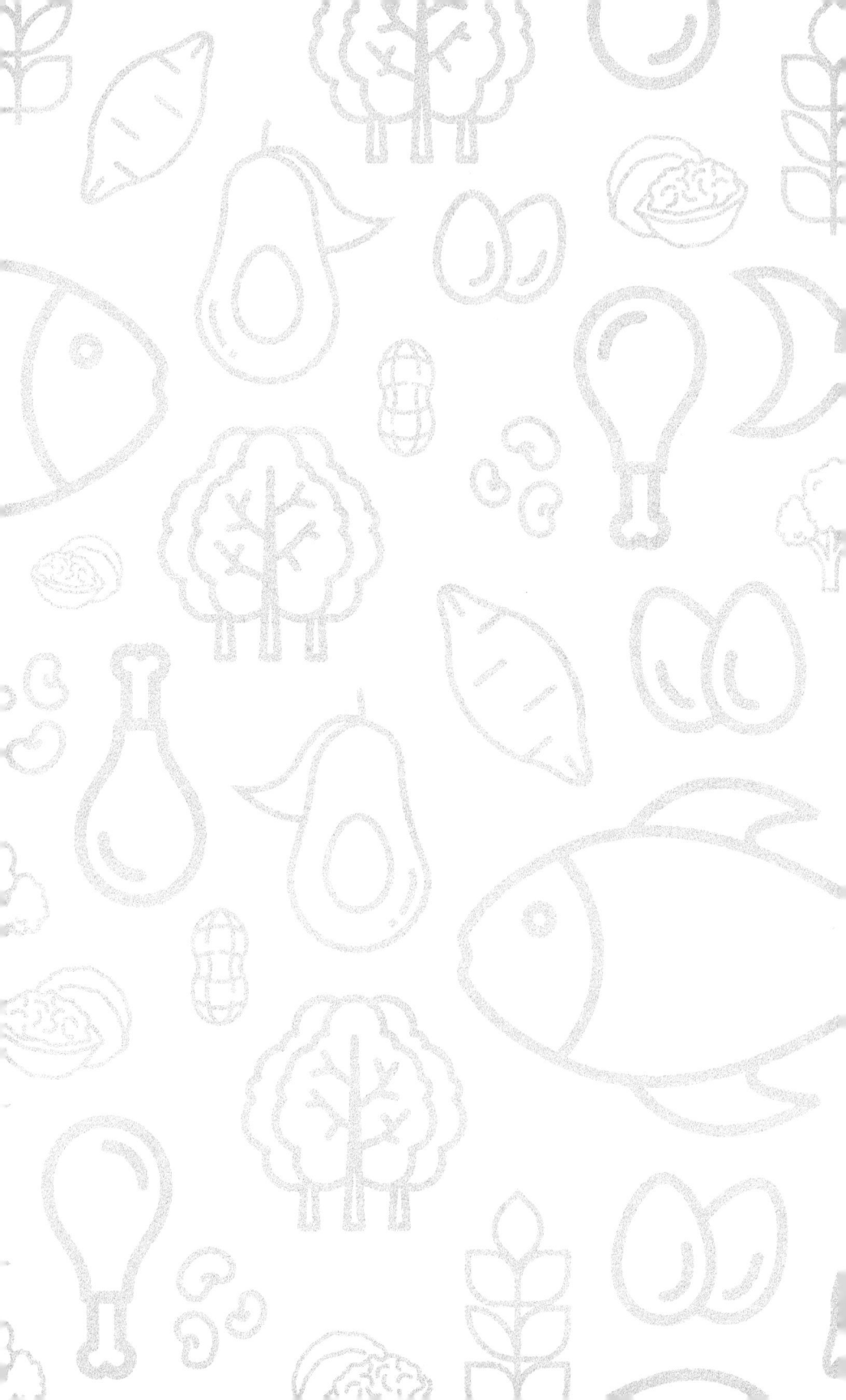

CHAPTER 15

Legumes, Nuts, Grains, and Seeds

L egumes, nuts, and grains share something in common with seeds: they are all seeds as well.

Seeds are great sources of fiber, several minerals, B vitamins, phytonutrients, and antioxidants. They are typically moderate in calories and protein and have very healthy fat profiles.

Legumes

Legumes are the seeds from the pods of certain plants. They include various beans, peas, and lentils. Legumes with high levels of nutrition are soybeans, chickpeas, lentils, green peas, pinto beans, kidney beans, black beans, and white beans.

A typical serving size varies from ½ to ⅔ cup depending on the legume. As a group, they are low in calories, low to moderate in protein, and contain both soluble and insoluble fiber. They also provide low amounts of natural sugar, and most are low in fats, except a few that are moderate in omega-3 ALA.

Legumes have a good vitamin profile, with high levels of vitamin B9 and moderate levels of B1 and B6.

They stand out nutritionally with their mineral profile. They have high levels of iron (moderate for women), and moderate to high amounts of magnesium, potassium, and zinc.

Soybeans are the legume with the best overall nutritional profile. In addition to the nutrients listed above, they provide high amounts of omega-6 and omega-3 ALA and have moderate to high levels of vitamins B2 and K as well as choline. They also include moderate levels of calcium and selenium.

Lastly, individual legumes contain the phytonutrients flavonoids (black beans and soybeans), carotenoids (green peas), and phytoestrogens (soybeans and soy products).

Nutrients vary by type of legume, so try to consume a variety to broaden your nutrient intake. As a group, they are an inexpensive and nutrient-dense food, earning their place on my top 10 list.

DYK

Legumes are the second most important food source in the world. There are over 20,000 different varieties.

Peanuts

I've placed peanuts between legumes and tree nuts intentionally. The reason is they are a legume, but their nutritional profile is more like a tree nut. Also, let's face it, most of us still consider them nuts.

While their nutrition is similar to a tree nut, peanuts cost significantly less on a per-ounce basis. In addition, dry roasted peanuts and peanut butter are very flexible foods that can be served as a healthy snack; added to meals, soups, or desserts; or even as a meal (peanut butter sandwiches).

The humble peanut is anything but nutritionally. By consuming ½ cup of dry roasted peanuts or 4½ tablespoons of peanut butter, you will be getting moderate levels of calories, protein, and fiber.

Peanuts also have a very good fat profile. Their saturated fat content is high, but this is offset by their very high levels of monounsaturated fats and omega-6 fatty acids. They have approximately 4 times the amount of unsaturated fats compared to saturated fats.

Their vitamin profile is excellent, with high amounts of vitamins B3, B6, and E, and moderate levels of B1, B2, B5, B9, and choline.

As for minerals, one serving of peanuts provides high levels of magnesium, zinc, phosphorus, manganese, and copper. In addition, you will receive moderate amounts of iron (men only), potassium, and selenium.

Peanuts contain the phytonutrients resveratrol and phenolic acids.

With their nutrient-dense profile, low cost, and great taste, peanuts are a great food option. Unless you have a peanut allergy, they are a fantastic addition to your diet.

Peanuts are on my top 10 list, which provides additional details about their nutritional profile.

Tree Nuts

These nuts are the seeds from certain trees. There are more than 20 types of edible tree nuts worldwide.

Nuts are a nutrient-dense food with healthy amounts of macronutrients, micronutrients, and phytonutrients. A serving size of one handful (30 grams) is low in calories (less than 10% of DRI), protein, carbohydrates, and natural sugars. In addition, most nuts have moderate amounts of fiber.

What makes nuts so nutritious is their moderate to high levels of monounsaturated fats and polyunsaturated omega-6 fats. Some are also high in omega-3 ALA. Their fat profile is incredibly healthy, with a ratio between 4:1 to 11:1 of unsaturated to saturated fats, depending on the nut. These fat profiles are among the best of all food groups.

Nuts also stand out nutritionally with their mineral content. They contain moderate to high levels of magnesium, iron (men only), and zinc. Nuts also contain moderate levels of a few B vitamins.

Nutritional values vary by nut. Below is a list of some of the most common nuts consumed in the U.S. Try eating a variety for better overall nutrition.

Almonds are one of the most nutritious nuts. Uniquely, they have high levels of vitamins E and B2. Almonds have the highest levels of magnesium. They also have the healthiest fat profile of all nuts.

Walnuts are another very healthy tree nut. They have the highest levels of omega-6 and omega-3 ALA (both above 75% of the DRI). They also have among the highest amounts of monounsaturated fats. Lastly, they have moderate levels of the vitamins B1 and B6. Walnuts contain the phytonutrients phenolic acids and phytoestrogens.

Cashews contain many of the same minerals as almonds and walnuts. They are the highest nut in vitamin K and minerals zinc, iron, and copper. Cashews contain phytonutrient phytoestrogens called lignans.

Pistachios have the highest levels of vitamins B1 and B6 and are high in both monounsaturated fats and omega-6. Pistachios contain phytonutrient carotenoids lutein and zeaxanthin.

Pecans have a similar nutritional profile to the nuts above, but with slightly lower levels. However, they have among the highest levels of monounsaturated fats, omega-6, and omega-3 ALA. They have the second-best fat profile among these nuts. Pecans contain phytonutrient flavonoids.

Nuts are a nutrient-dense food group and on my top 10 list of nutrient-dense foods.

Whole Grains

Whole grains are the seeds of grasses. Some of the most common whole-grain foods in the U.S. include whole wheat, quinoa, long grain brown rice, corn, and oats.

Whole-grain kernels are comprised of three parts: the outer shell, called the bran; a sprouting section of seed, called the germ; and an energy supply, called the endosperm. All three provide important but different nutrients. You are not getting the full nutritional benefit of grain foods if they are not "whole," with all three parts present.

🔍 DYK

For thousands of years, grains have been the most prevalent carbohydrate for humans. Rice, corn (dry and ground), and wheat make up most grain consumption. Today, the world's population gets approximately half of its daily calories from grain foods.

Per serving, whole grains are typically low in calories, protein, fats, carbohydrates, and natural sugar. The nutrient content of whole-grain foods can vary significantly, so it's healthy to eat a variety. Below is a description of the most common U.S. grain foods.

100% whole-grain wheat bread and quinoa are the most nutritious grain foods and are nutrient-dense. They provide a broad set of nutrients at healthy levels and have similar nutritional profiles. A serving size of whole-wheat bread (two slices) contains moderate levels of protein, fiber, and the polyunsaturated fats omega-6 and omega-3 ALA.

One serving of quinoa (¾ cup) has slightly less protein and fiber, but similar levels of fats.

Both grain foods have excellent fat profiles with 3–6 times the amount of unsaturated fats compared to saturated fats.

In terms of vitamin profile, whole-wheat bread and quinoa contain moderate to high levels of vitamins B1, B2, B5, B6, and B9. Whole-wheat bread also has high levels of vitamins B3 and E.

In addition, both have high levels of magnesium, iron (moderate for women), phosphorus, copper, and manganese, and moderate levels of zinc. Whole-wheat bread further has moderate amounts of calcium and selenium. Note that whole-grain rye bread is full of many of the same nutrients as 100% whole-wheat bread.

Both of these grain foods contain the phytonutrient carotenoids, lutein and zeaxanthin, and phenolic acids.

100% whole-wheat bread and quinoa are the two grain foods that are nutrient-dense and are on my top 10 list of the most nutritious foods.

Long-grain brown rice is also a highly nutritious grain food. It has several of the same nutrients as whole wheat and quinoa, but at lower levels. Again, make sure you select whole-grain products when choosing your rice. This will increase the protein, B vitamins, and mineral levels.

Corn and oats are not nutrient-dense foods, but they do contain moderate levels of several important minerals and soluble fiber (more so in oats) and B vitamins and insoluble fiber (more so in corn). These are healthy additions to your diet when in their whole-grain forms.

Seeds

Seeds are not an item typically thought of as a common food source. However, they are very nutritious.

The seeds in this section are even more nutrient dense per gram than legumes, nuts, and grains. The seeds from chia, flax, pumpkin, and cacao plants are easily added to salads, smoothies, cereals, oatmeal, soups, or other dishes. Most of them have a very mild flavor profile, so you likely won't taste them when added (except cacao, which has a slight chocolate flavor).

These seeds provide healthy amounts of many important minerals, unsaturated fats, fiber, and phytonutrients. They are all low in calories, protein, and natural sugars.

Chia seeds are chock full of minerals. Two daily tablespoons provide high levels of fiber, magnesium, iron (moderate for women), phosphorus, manganese, copper, and selenium. They also have moderate amounts of calcium and zinc.

In addition, chia seeds contain moderate levels of vitamins B1 and B2. They are also very high in omega-3 ALA (over 100% of DRI) and moderate in omega-6. Lastly, they are a good source of the phytonutrients phenolic acids and flavonoids.

Pro Move

Soaking your chia seeds increases their bioavailability (absorption and use by the body). They only need approximately 20 minutes or can be soaked overnight. Refrigerate them to increase their shelf life.

Flax seeds provide many of the same nutrients as chia seeds but at slightly lower levels. Two daily tablespoons provide very high levels of omega-3 ALA, and moderate levels of magnesium, iron (men only), phosphorus, manganese, and selenium. They also have moderate levels of fiber and contain the phytonutrient lignans.

Pro Move

Enhance your flax seeds bioavailability by grinding them (a coffee grinder will do this). Once ground, keep them in the refrigerator. Soaking these seeds may also improve bioavailability.

Pumpkin seeds are another very healthy seed full of minerals. Two daily tablespoons of pumpkin seeds have most of the same levels of minerals as chia seeds (in some cases higher). The exceptions are calcium and selenium, which are present at lower levels.

Pumpkin seeds have high levels of omega-6 and moderate levels of monounsaturated fats.

Note that pumpkin seeds are often sold as "pepitas," with the shell removed. This lowers their fiber content, but the rest of the nutrients are approximately the same. They are also sold raw or roasted. Both are nutritious and it appears raw has a higher vitamin and mineral content, but lower phytonutrient content. As with chia seeds, bioavailability can be increased by soaking them.

Cacao powder is made from the seeds of the cacao tree, just like chocolate. Cacao powder is more nutritious than cocoa powder because it is roasted at lower temperatures, but the taste is more bitter. When added to foods, it has a chocolate flavor, but not as strongly as cocoa powder.

Cacao powder is a nutritional powerhouse. Two tablespoons have similar mineral levels to chia seeds but are higher in important iron (significantly higher), magnesium, and potassium. Cacao powder is also higher in monounsaturated fats, but lower than chia seeds in fiber, vitamin B1, zinc, and omega-6.

There are several other seeds that also have high amounts of minerals and phytonutrient levels. These include sesame, sunflower, and hemp seeds. Give your diet a nutritional boost by adding some of these to your meals.

With their high nutritional density, chia, flax, and pumpkin seeds make my honorable mention list of nutrient-dense foods. I left cacao powder off the list of top seeds as I have read that some versions are high in saturated fat.

My Plant-Based Food Approach

My overall dietary strategy for plant-based foods is to consume many different types daily with a focus on the most nutritious. I eat plant foods in whole form at all three meals, focusing on fresh, frozen, and canned unprocessed versions.

My weekly go-to plant foods include broccoli (often as broccoli rice), spinach, carrots, avocados, berries, oranges, lemons, apples, sweet peppers, tomatoes (and tomato sauce), bananas, peanut butter, almonds, walnuts, whole-grain bread, tea, coffee, and several different types of seeds.

On average, I eat 15–20 different plant foods per day, spanning all of the different plant food groups described above. The amounts I consume are often lower than typical serving sizes. This allows me to get a wider variety of different types without consuming too much food.

I know this sounds like a lot of plant foods, but if you regularly consume vegetables, fruits, grains, legumes, nuts, and seeds in your diet, it adds up quickly. Also, teas and coffee count towards this total.

My cheat code to getting these higher levels is to focus on bowl meals. Examples of these meals are oatmeal, breakfast cereals, salads, smoothies, chilis, etc. These meals are described in more detail in the last section of the book.

My plant-food selections help me attain healthy daily levels of complex carbohydrates, fiber, unsaturated fats (except omega-3 EPA/DHA), all vitamins (except D and B12), and several priority minerals. They also provide a variety of several different phytonutrients.

📖 Organic Foods Facts Break

Is it worth buying organic food?

➜ *Certified organic foods have restrictions on how plant or animal foods are grown or raised. These restrictions include the use of pesticides, fertilizers, hormones for growth, antibiotics, and the type of feed. For USDA Organic certification, there are strict standards, and you should look for this certification on your food packaging.*

➜ *The positive aspects of organic foods are the lower exposure to chemicals, hormones, and antibiotics. While the science is not comprehensive on the health benefits, it is generally believed that organic foods lower the risk of long-term health problems.*

➜ *The negatives of organic foods are their higher expense (costing between 10–50% more), the fact that they may not significantly reduce health risks, and that organic food doesn't have higher nutrient levels than non-organic.*

➜ *If you decide to buy organic food, reduce costs by buying frozen vegetables and fruits or buying in bulk. Also, focus on buying organic foods known to be high in pesticides, such as strawberries, spinach, kale, apples, grapes, peppers, pears, and green beans.*

➜ *If you decide not to buy organic, you can remove pesticides on the skins of your plant foods by soaking your foods in water with baking soda for 15–20 minutes. Studies show a 60–90% reduction in pesticides using this method.*

➜ *Lastly, don't be fooled by the food labels "natural" or "locally grown." This is no guarantee that the food is organic.*

Additional sources used for legumes, nuts, grains, and seeds description: [200] [201] [202] [203] [204] [205] [206] [207] [208] [209] [210] [211] [212]

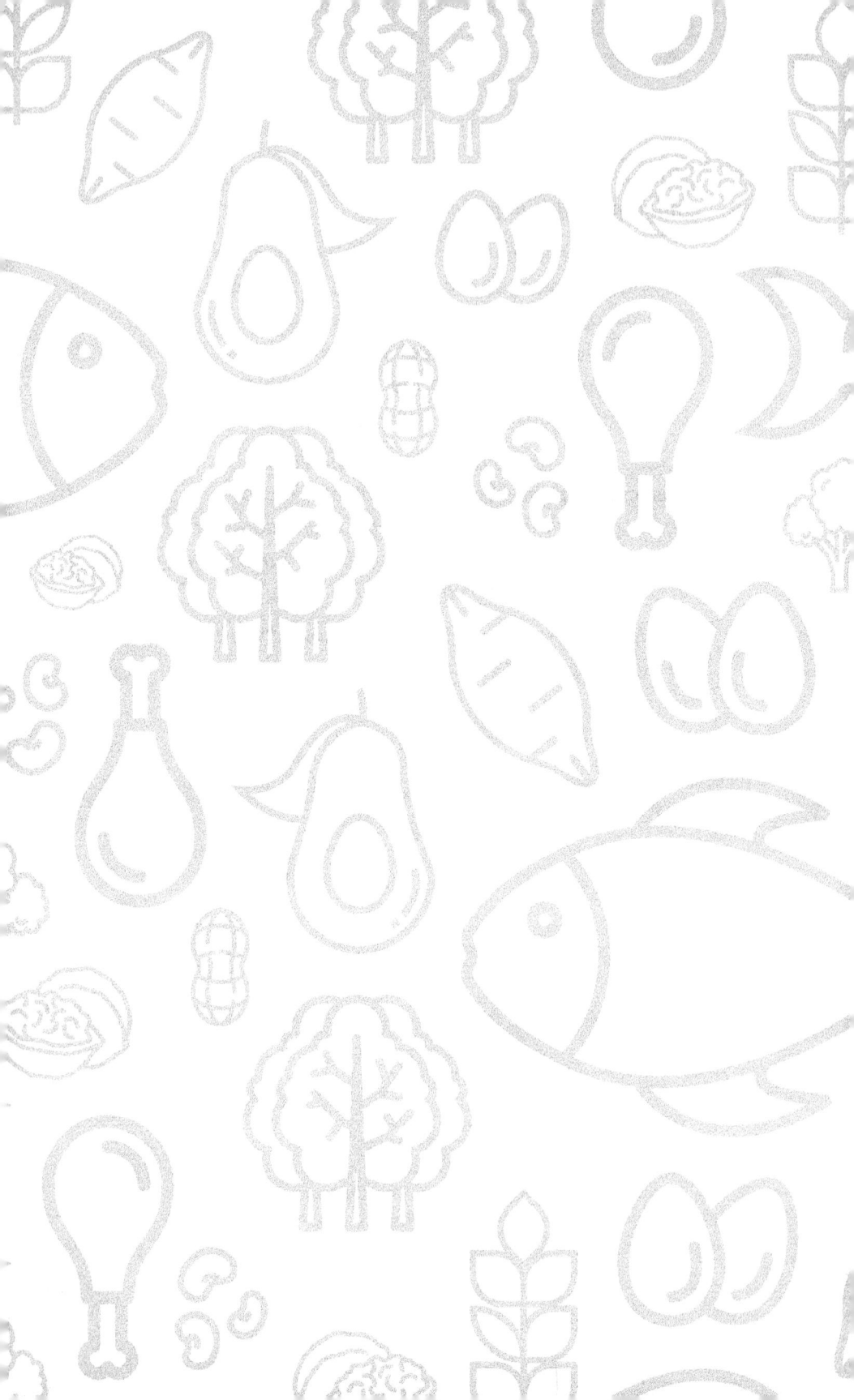

CHAPTER 16

Top 10 Nutrient-Dense Foods and Honorable Mentions

A s you saw in the last few chapters, there are many nutritious foods. This chapter focuses on those with the *highest* level of nutrition, what I call the "Top 10 Nutrient-Dense Foods." I've also included a number of "Honorable Mention Foods."

I recommend you add most, if not all, of these foods to your diet. If you include them regularly, then you greatly increase your odds of consuming a fully nutritious diet.

For each food or group listed below, I provide a summary of its nutrient profile, health benefits, and dietary considerations. Additionally, I have included a chart for each food or group, showing where it has healthy levels of important nutrients.

There is a lot of information here; don't worry about memorizing it. My goal is for this chapter to become a good reference for your future food questions. In tandem with the book's last section containing example meals, I hope these are helpful to you in building a healthy diet.

As a reminder, a food contains "very high" levels of a nutrient when it provides 50% or more of the daily benchmark, "high" levels when providing 20–49%, "moderate" at 10–19%, "low" at less than 10%.

Lastly, my recommendation is to consume on average at least one to two of these top foods at every meal, in typical serving sizes. When making my meals at home, I try to average about six to eight of these foods daily (top 10 and honorable mention foods).

Top 10 Nutrient-Dense Foods

1. Salmon

Background: Farmed Atlantic, wild pink, and wild sockeye salmon are the most consumed in the U.S. A serving size is 6 ounces.

Nutrient summary: These salmon provide high levels of protein and unsaturated fats. One of the few foods with very high levels of omega-3 EPA/DHA. They have excellent vitamin, mineral and fat profiles.

Health benefits: Studies show regular consumption significantly improves cardiovascular, bone and brain health, and reduce the risk of depression, Alzheimer's, and inflammation.

Dietary considerations: Canned and bulk frozen fillet salmon are cheaper than fresh fillets. With canned, try to ensure no sodium is added.

Salmon, 6-ounces

Macronutrients	DRI Level	Vitamins	DRI Level	Minerals	DRI Level
Calories:	~235-350	A	**Moderate	Priority:	
Protein:	High	B1	**Very High	Magnesium	Moderate
Fats:		B2	High	Potassium	High
Saturated	**Moderate	B3	Very High	Iron	*Mod/Low
Monounsaturated	Moderate	B5	High	Zinc	***Moderate
Omega-3 ALA	**Moderate	B6	High	Calcium	***High
Omega-3 EPA /DHA	Very High	B9	**Moderate	Others:	
Unsat/ Saturated Ratio:	3:1 Very Good	B12	Very High	Phosphorus	Very High
		D	Very High	Copper	Moderate
		E	Moderate	Selenium	Very High
		Choline	High		

Source: USDA Food Data Central
DRI Level Scale: Very high: 50%+, High: 20-49%, Moderate: 10-19%
*Men/Women   **Farmed Atlantic Salmon only   ***Canned Pink and Sockeye only

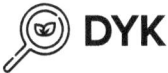

⊚ DYK

Is farmed or wild caught salmon healthier? Both are very healthy. Farmed Atlantic salmon is higher in unsaturated fats and has a slightly better fat profile. Wild caught salmon is higher in calcium, iron, and zinc. They have similar protein and vitamin levels, and both are low in mercury. Try to select farmed fish that originates from the U.S., Canada, or Norway. These countries have higher standards on antibiotic use.

2. Chicken 🍗

Background: Breasts and thighs are the most popular poultry cuts in the U.S. A typical serving size is 6 ounces.

Nutrient summary: These cuts of chicken provide high levels of protein and have a good fat ratio at approximately 2:1. Both have moderate to high levels of several important vitamins and minerals.

Health benefits: Poultry is associated with a lower risk of certain chronic conditions. It also contains tryptophan, which is linked to higher levels of serotonin. Serotonin is believed to be good for our brains in several ways, supporting memory and happiness. It can also improve sleep quality.

Dietary considerations: Chicken preparation has a big impact on its health benefits/risks. When deep fried, rotisserie, or processed as deli meat, it is higher in calories, saturated fats, and sodium.

Chicken (6-ounces)

Macronutrients	DRI Level	Vitamins	DRI Level	Minerals	DRI Level
Calories:	~280-360	B1	**Mod/ Very High	Priority:	
Protein:	**Very High/ High	B2	**Mod/High	Magnesium	Moderate
Fats:		B3	Very High	Potassium	Moderate
Saturated	**Low/High	B5	High	Iron	*High/Mod
Monounsaturated	**Low/High	B6	Very High	Zinc	**Mod/High
Omega-6	**Low/High	B12	High	Others:	
Omega-3 ALA	**Low/High	K	**Low/High	Phosphorous	High
Unsat/ Saturated Ratio:	2:1 Good	Choline	High	Copper	Moderate
				Selenium	Very High

Source: USDA Food Data Central
DRI Level Scale: Very high: 50%+, High: 20-49%, Moderate: 10-19%
*Men/Women   **Breasts/Thighs

3. Chicken Eggs ⟮⟯

Background: Chicken eggs are the most widely consumed eggs in the world. The serving size is 2 eggs.

Nutrient summary: Eggs have moderate amounts of protein and several unsaturated fats. The fat ratio is a healthy 2:1. They provide healthy levels of several vitamins and priority minerals.

Health benefits: Eggs are high in dietary cholesterol, but several studies show most people do not absorb high levels of this cholesterol and suggest it is not linked to increased LDL or high triglyceride blood levels. In fact, eggs have been found to increase HDL (good cholesterol) blood levels.

Dietary considerations: Unless you are at risk for cardiovascular health issues, you may consider going up to three eggs for meals. This would raise the protein and several nutrient levels. If you consume eggs daily, then it may be best to limit yourself to two.

Eggs, two

Macronutrients	DRI Level	Vitamins	DRI Level	Minerals	DRI Level
Calories:	~**150/225	A	High	**Priority:**	
Protein:	Moderate	B2	High	Iron	*High/Mod
Fats:		B5	High	Zinc	Moderate
Saturated	Moderate	B6	**Mod/High	**Others:**	
Monounsaturated	Moderate	B9	Moderate	Phosphorous	High
Omega-6	**Mod/High	B12	**High/Very High	Copper	***Moderate
Omega-3 ALA	Moderate	D	Moderate	Selenium	Very High
Unsat/Saturated Ratio:	2:1 Good	E	***Moderate		
		K	***Moderate		
		Choline	Very High		

Source: USDA Food Data Central   DRI Level Scale: Very high: 50%+, High: 20-49%, Moderate: 10-19%

*Men/Women   **2 Eggs/3 Eggs   ***3 Eggs Only

4. Cooked Broccoli and Kale 🥦 🥬

Background: Calabrese broccoli is the most common U.S. variety, with a typical serving of 1 cup.

Nutrient summary: Cooked broccoli and kale offer moderate fiber and very little fat aside from omega-3 ALA. Their main value comes from high vitamin and mineral levels.

Health benefits: Both contain glucosinolates—organosulfur compounds shown to support immune function and reduce inflammation, with antiviral, antibacterial, and potentially anticancer properties.

Dietary considerations: Excellent as a side or added to bowl meals. If you dislike broccoli, frozen "broccoli rice" has comparable nutrients and can be easily mixed into soups or chilis without affecting flavor.

Cooked Broccoli and Kale, 1 cup

Macronutrients	DRI Level	Vitamins	DRI Level	Minerals	DRI Level
Calories:	~50	A	**Mod/High	Priority:	
Protein:	Low	B2	Moderate	Magnesium	Moderate
Fats:		B5	***Moderate	Potassium	***Moderate
Omega-3 ALA	**Moderate/ High	B6	***High	Iron	*Mod/Low
Unsat/ Saturated Ratio:	2.5-4:1 Very Good	B9	High	Calcium	****High
Total Carbohydrates:	Low	C	**Very High /High	Others:	
Fiber:	Moderate	E	Moderate	Phosphorous	***Moderate
		K	Very High	Copper	Moderate
				Manganese	**Mod/High

Source: USDA Food Data Central
DRI Level Scale: Very high: 50%+, High: 20-49%, Moderate: 10-19%
*Men/Women   **Broccoli/Kale   ***Broccoli Only   ****Kale Only

5. Avocados 🥑

Background: Mexico is the biggest producer of avocados worldwide, and the U.S. currently gets most of its avocados from there. The serving size is 1 medium avocado.

Nutrient summary: Avocados are one of the few fruits that are high in unsaturated fats and fiber. While they are moderate in saturated fats, avocados' overall fat ratio is an excellent 5:1 and can help with your diet's overall fat profile. They have an excellent vitamin profile and a very good mineral profile.

Health benefits: Studies associate regular consumption of avocados with normal blood pressure, immune system health, heart and brain health, and cancer prevention.

Dietary considerations: This fruit is easy to use in sandwiches, salads, or dips (guacamole), and pairs well with several entrees. At 240 calories, it is calorie rich, so I always buy smaller versions. If concerned, consider consuming only ½ the avocado. Even at half size, this is a very nutritious food.

Avocado, 1 medium

Macronutrients	DRI Level	Vitamins	DRI Level	Minerals	DRI Level
Calories:	~240	B1	Moderate	Priority:	
Protein:	Low	B2	Moderate	Magnesium	Moderate
Fats:		B3	Moderate	Potassium	High
Saturated	Moderate	B5	High	Iron	*Mod/Low
Monounsaturated	High	B6	High	Zinc	Moderate
Omega-6	Moderate	B9	High	Others:	
Omega-3 ALA	Moderate	C	Moderate	Phosphorus	Moderate
Unsat/ Saturated Ratio:	5:1 Excellent	K	Moderate	Manganese	Moderate
Total Carbohydrates:	Low				
Fiber	High				

Source: USDA Food Data Central

DRI Level Scale: Very high: 50%+, High: 20-49%, Moderate: 10-19%   *Men/Women*

6. Sweet Potatoes

Background: Sweet potatoes are originally from Central and South America. A typical serving size is 1 medium sweet potato with skin.

Nutrient summary: Sweet potatoes contain moderate amounts of soluble and insoluble fiber. They have healthy amounts of many important vitamins and minerals.

Health benefits: Studies show that consuming sweet potatoes is associated with several potential health benefits for our gut microbiota, eyes, skin, and immune systems.

Dietary considerations: Sweet potatoes have moderate amounts of natural sugar but when eaten with the skin, their fiber helps reduce blood sugar spikes and provides more nutrients. Try to avoid adding butter and brown sugar to your sweet potato, as it increases the simple sugar and saturated fat levels and calorie count. Sweet potatoes taste great on their own.

If you are wondering about sweet potato fries, these can also be a healthy option. Bake or air fry them, as these cooking methods retain many of the natural nutrients in sweet potatoes. If you put oil on them, try to use olive oil, as it adds more healthy nutrients to the fries.

Sweet Potato, 1 medium with skin

Macronutrients	DRI Level	Vitamins	DRI Level	Minerals	DRI Level
Calories:	~100	A	Very High	Priority:	
Protein:	Low	B1	Moderate	Magnesium	Moderate
Total Carbohydrates:	Low	B2	Moderate	Potassium	Moderate
Natural Sugar	Moderate	B3	Moderate	Iron	*Mod/Low
Fiber	Moderate	B5	High	Others:	
		B6	High	Phosphorous	Moderate
		C	High	Copper	High
				Manganese	High

Source: USDA Food Data Central
DRI Level Scale: Very high: 50%+, High: 20-49%, Moderate: 10-19%   *Men/Women

7. Legumes

Background: Nutritious legumes include soybeans, chickpeas, lentils, green peas, pinto beans, kidney beans, black beans, and white beans. A serving size is ½ to ⅔ cup, depending on the legume.

Nutrient summary: Legumes are high in fiber. They are generally low in most fats, but soybeans are uniquely high in unsaturated fats. Most legumes have a good vitamin profile, and soybeans have an even better one. Legumes' most impressive nutritional asset is their mineral content, as they have moderate to high levels of almost all priority minerals.

Health benefits: Studies show legumes help reduce cardiovascular risk, lower LDL levels, and raise HDL levels. They may also reduce the risk of type 2 diabetes and improve weight management. High soluble and insoluble fiber levels in legumes are good for gut and digestive tract health.

Dietary considerations: Legumes are not very popular in the U.S., but please consider adding them into your diet. If reluctant, try them in soups or chilis, or make them into a dip like hummus.

Legumes, ½- ⅔ cup

Macronutrients	DRI Level	Vitamins	DRI Level	Minerals	DRI Level
Calories:	~85-170	B1	Moderate	Priority:	
Protein:	Moderate	B2	**High	Magnesium	***High/Mod
Fats:		B5	**Moderate	Potassium	Moderate
Omega-6	**High	B6	Moderate	Iron	*High/Mod
Omega-3 ALA	***High/Mod	B9	***Mod/ High	Zinc	Moderate
Unsat/ Saturated Ratio:	2-6:1 Good/ Excellent	K	**Moderate	Calcium	**High
Total Carbohydrates:	Low	Choline	**Moderate	Others:	
Fiber	High			Phosphorus	High
				Copper	High
				Manganese	High
				Selenium	**High

Source: USDA Food Data Central
DRI Level Scale: Very high: 50%+, High: 20-49%, Moderate: 10-19%
*Men/Women   **Soy Products only   ***Soy Products/Other Legumes

8. Roasted Peanuts and Peanut Butter 🥜

Background: Under U.S. law, any product labeled peanut butter must be made almost completely from peanuts. A serving size is ½ cup roasted peanuts or 4.5 tablespoons of peanut butter.

Nutrient summary: Peanuts and peanut butter are very similar nutritionally. They have healthy levels of protein and fiber, and an excellent fat profile at a ratio of 4:1. This is another food that can help your diet's overall fat profile. They also have a great vitamin profile, especially with B vitamins and E. Their mineral profile is very good as well, with healthy levels of several.

Health benefits: Peanuts are associated in many studies with lower cardiovascular risk, lower overall mortality, reduced LDL and triglyceride levels, a lower risk of diabetes, and better weight management.

Dietary considerations: This is a very nutritious food. However, make sure to limit your peanut consumption to the serving sizes listed here, as peanuts are calorie dense. Also, be careful to avoid peanut products with high levels of sodium and sugar added.

Peanuts and Peanut Butter, ½ cup and 4 ½ tablespoons

Macronutrients	DRI Level	Vitamins	DRI Level	Minerals	DRI Level
Calories:	~440	B1	Moderate	**Priority:**	
Protein:	Moderate	B2	Moderate	Magnesium	High
Fats:		B3	Very High	Potassium	Moderate
Saturated	High	B5	Moderate	Iron	*Mod/Low
Monounsaturated	Very High	B6	High	Zinc	High
Omega-6	Very High	B9	Moderate	**Others:**	
Unsat/ Saturated Ratio:	4:1 Excellent	E	High	Phosphorus	High
Total Carbohydrates:	Low	Choline	Moderate	Copper	High
Fiber	Moderate			Manganese	Very High
				Selenium	Moderate

Source: USDA Food Data Central
DRI Level Scale: Very high: 50%+, High: 20-49%, Moderate: 10-19%   *Men/Women

9. Tree Nuts 🥜

Background: Some of the most nutritious tree nuts include almonds, walnuts, cashews, pistachios, and pecans. One serving size is a handful or 30 grams or 1 ounce.

Nutrient summary: Tree nuts have an excellent fat profile. The unsaturated to saturated ratio is approximately 4:1 to 11:1, depending on the nut. This is another food group that can help improve your overall diet fat profile. In addition, nuts have moderate to high levels of several important minerals. They have a modest vitamin profile.

Health benefits: Several credible studies show that tree nuts lower inflammation, reduce the risk of cardiovascular disease, and decrease the risk of diabetes, especially in women.

Dietary considerations: Like peanuts, tree nuts are a calorie dense food, so be careful with portion sizes. Some studies show that high nut serving sizes do not lead to weight gain, but I recommend being cautious about consuming too much.

Lastly, as with peanuts, you need to be careful about additives in tree nut products. Added sodium and sugar are the main concerns.

Tree Nuts, a handful or 30 grams

Macronutrients	DRI Level	Vitamins	DRI Level	Minerals	DRI Level
Calories:	~170-200	B1	Moderate	Priority:	
Protein:	Low	B2	**High	Magnesium	Moderate
Fats:		B6	Moderate	Iron	*Mod/Low
Monounsaturated	High	E	**High	Zinc	Moderate
Omega-6	High	K	****Moderate	Others:	
Omega-3 ALA	***Very High			Phosphorus	High
Unsat/ Saturated Ratio:	4-11:1 Excellent			Copper	High
Total Carbohydrates:	Low			Manganese	Moderate
Fiber	Moderate				

Source: USDA Food Data Central
DRI Level Scale: Very high: 50%+, High: 20-49%, Moderate: 10-19%
*Men/Women   **Almonds Only   ***Walnuts Only   ****Cashews Only

10. 100% Whole-Wheat Bread and Quinoa 🌾

Background: A serving size is 2 slices of whole-wheat bread or ¾ cup of quinoa. Quinoa is one of the few plant foods providing all nine essential amino acids.

Nutrient summary: These grain foods have moderate amounts of fiber and an excellent fat profile. They have moderate levels of the unsaturated fats omega-6 and omega-3 ALA fatty acids. Their primary nutritional value comes from their outstanding vitamin profile, with moderate to high levels of several B vitamins. Whole-wheat bread also has a moderate amount of vitamin E. In addition, whole-wheat bread and quinoa are moderate to high in several priority minerals.

Health benefits: Studies show that regular whole grain consumption reduces the risk of several chronic conditions, including type 2 diabetes, high blood pressure, high cholesterol, and certain cancers.

Dietary considerations: Be careful when selecting your breads, as many products present themselves as whole wheat by using terms like "cracked wheat" or "multi-grain," but do not use 100% of the whole grain. They also often add unhealthy levels of sodium and/or sugar.

100% Whole-wheat Bread and Quinoa, 2 slices and ¾ cup

Macronutrients	DRI Level	Vitamins	DRI Level	Minerals	DRI Level
Calories:	~180-250	B1	***High/ Mod	Priority:	
Protein:	**Moderate	B2	Moderate	Magnesium	High
Fats:		B3	**High	Iron	*High/Mod
Omega-6	Moderate	B5	Moderate	Zinc	Moderate
Omega-3 ALA	Moderate	B6	Moderate	Calcium	**Moderate
Unsat/ Saturated Ratio:	3-7:1 Excellent	B9	Moderate	Others:	
Total Carbohydrates:	Moderate	E	**Moderate	Phosphorus	High
Fiber	Moderate			Copper	High
				Manganese	Very High
				Selenium	**High

Source: USDA Food Data Central

DRI Level Scale: Very high: 50%+, High: 20-49%, Moderate: 10-19%

*Men/Women   **Whole Wheat Only   ***Whole Wheat/Quinoa

Honorable Mention Nutrient-Dense Foods

Sardines, Tuna, and Rainbow Trout

Background: A serving size of 6 ounces is 200–300 calories.

Nutrient summary: These fatty fish have very similar nutrients to salmon. They are high in protein and have a good fat profile at a ratio of 2:1 unsaturated to saturated fats or better. Most are very high in omega-3 EPA/DHA. They are all rich in several vitamins and most priority minerals.

Sardines are the nutrient leader of this group with an excellent 5.5:1 fat ratio. They are the highest in omega-3 ALA, omega-6, and monounsaturated fats.

Health benefits: Similar to salmon's.

Dietary considerations: All these fish are great alternatives to salmon. Note that tuna fillets can be expensive, so consider buying canned which is much cheaper with the same or very similar nutrient levels. When selecting your canned tuna, try using "skipjack," sometimes called "light" or "chunk light" for the lowest mercury levels. Also, make sure it has healthy levels of vitamin D and no sodium added. This information should be on the nutrient facts label.

Blueberries, Strawberries, Blackberries, Raspberries, and Kiwis

Background: A serving size of 1 cup (or 1 kiwi) is 50–85 calories.

Nutrient summary: These are not a nutrient-dense food group from a macro and micronutrient perspective. However, they do have a decent vitamin profile and are a great source of vitamin C. Also, they provide healthy levels of fiber.

Berries' nutrient superpower is their high levels of phytonutrients with antioxidants and anti-inflammatories. They have high levels of a flavonoid called anthocyanidins, several subclasses of phenolic acids, and the phytoestrogens lignans and resveratrol.

Health benefits: Studies show berries' phytonutrients (and vitamin C levels) may help reduce the risks of cancer, cardiovascular disease, diabetes, and cognitive decline, in addition to improving overall immune system health.

Dietary considerations: Currently, there is a "love affair" with blueberries because they are the most studied berry. These are delicious berries, but don't ignore strawberries, blackberries, raspberries, or kiwis. They all offer as many, if not more, nutritional benefits as blueberries. Eat a variety to get the full benefit of berries.

Also, try to eat kiwis with the skins, which contain several nutrients and fiber. If the texture turns you off, then try them in a smoothie.

Chia, Flax, and Pumpkin Seeds

Background: A serving size of 2 tablespoons is 75–120 calories.

Nutrient summary: These seeds all have great fat profiles and can be a nutritional boost to meals by adding high levels of unsaturated fats with low levels of saturated fat. They have an excellent 4:1 to 7:1 fat ratio. They also will significantly increase the levels of several priority minerals in your diet.

These seeds provide many phytonutrients. Chia seeds have the phenolic acids caffeic, quercetin, and kaempferol. Flax seeds contain high levels of lignans. Pumpkin seeds contain different carotenoids, phenolic acids, and phytoestrogens.

Health benefits: Studies indicate that these seeds may help reduce LDL levels and lower the risk of type 2 diabetes. In addition, they may help with inflammation and cancer risk.

Dietary considerations: These seeds can easily be included in salads, oatmeal, smoothies, or soups. They do not have a strong flavor, so you will barely notice them in your foods.

Final Section Thoughts

With this background on the most nutritious foods, let's now move on to the final section. Rather than being redundant, I provide the key takeaways from this section at the beginning of the next section. In it, I describe developing dietary goals and how to build healthy meals all with foods described in this section.

These descriptions include the most nutritious animal foods and plant-based foods and the number of these foods to target on a daily or weekly basis.

Additional sources used for top food descriptions: [213] [214] [215] [216] [217] [218] [219] [220] [221] [222] [223] [224] [225] [226] [227] [228] [229] [230]

Absolute Nutritious Meals

With your new understanding of the most nutritious foods, let's now jump into how you can use these foods to build great meals. In this section, I have developed several meals that provide incredibly high levels of nutrition. As with the foods recommended, these are neither exotic nor gourmet meals. No, these are simple-to-make, delicious dishes that many of us grew up eating and won't break your budget.

Before getting into the meals, let's establish some approaches that will help make your new diet a success. First, I recommend you have a defined strategy for your nutritional goals. You should also have a healthy dieting perspective to increase your chances of sticking to it. Lastly, I suggest some strategies that will help keep your meals high in important nutrients and moderate in those that are unhealthy at high levels.

Dietary Nutritional Goals

I believe a primary goal for each of us should be to achieve absolute nutrition on a daily basis. This is probably not shocking if you've read the other sections. What does absolute nutrition mean? Simply put, consuming daily meals that provide the recommended levels of essential macronutrients and micronutrients.

A second important goal for your diet is to limit certain nutrients and added ingredients to no more than recommended daily levels. The ones to limit are added sugar, sodium, and saturated fat. Again, this is not surprising given this book's other recommendations. As you know by now, high levels of these nutrients greatly increase your risk of significant health issues.

Accomplishing both these goals can help you lead a long and healthy life.

A Healthy Perspective on Diet, Excluding Perfection

Sticking to a healthy diet is difficult. It takes commitment. However, you should not beat yourself up if you stray every now and then. Dieting should not feel like a prison sentence.

Remember that nothing in life is perfect. If you expect perfection with your diet, you are almost assured disappointment. Nutritional perfection every day would be asking too much. This is one of the reasons more than half of the people who start diets stop within a year and lose any health benefits gained.

This is just the reality of having busy lives full of other priorities like jobs, kids, parents, friends, and the need to have some fun and reduce stress. Your diet approach needs to be balanced with these priorities.

I believe establishing this expectation up front will help you better adhere to your diet and be more satisfied with it. While you should not aim for perfection, you should consistently follow your diet. Otherwise, you will not achieve your nutritional and good health goals. My suggestion is that you focus on sticking to your diet at least five days a week. This gives you a couple of days off every week.

When you do take that break, please try to still use some of the strategies listed below and continue to consume my recommended foods. On your off days, you may not achieve 100% full nutrition, but if you reach 50–75% of most essential nutrients that's not a bad nutritional day. Also, during your hiatus, try to limit your portion sizes of foods high in saturated fat, added sugar, and sodium.

If you are worried or feel guilty about taking a day off, take some comfort in the fact that humans did not evolve in a perfect nutritional environment. Undoubtedly, our ancestors consumed varied levels of nutrients on a day-to-day basis. This is likely why excess amounts of most nutrients are stored for short periods of time by the body for future needs.

Daily Calories and Weight

We are a society obsessed with weight. However, studies show that low body weight is not necessarily the best priority for good health. In fact, studies have found that being moderately overweight (not obese) can be healthier than very thin. This is particularly true for the elderly, for whom being moderately overweight seems to lower mortality and have a potentially preventative effect against certain diseases.

Even with these health findings, I realize many people think that weight and calories are important factors when considering diet. If you are interested in knowing your specific daily caloric target and other nutrients, you can use the U.S. Department of Agriculture's DRI Calculator Results. It uses your age, sex, weight, height, and activity level as a basis to calculate a daily calorie estimate.

The link is *https://www.nal.usda.gov/human-nutrition-and-food-safety/dri-calculator*. One suggestion for using this tool: Use your ideal body weight, not necessarily your current weight, for the calculations. In other words, if you are 160 pounds and you think a good weight for you is 145 pounds, enter 145 pounds. This will provide more accurate results for your nutritional needs.

Also note that the daily protein and carbohydrate recommendations from this tool are not consistent with my recommendations. I explain the reasons for my recommended levels of these nutrients in Section 2 if you are interested.

Even with different ages and sizes, most of us are in a daily calorie range of 2,000–3,000. A healthy weight will likely be maintained if you're active, eat whole, unprocessed foods and keep daily calorie intake within this range.

If you are not interested in using the tool, don't worry. The daily calorie average for the meal examples described below is 1,900, slightly less than most people's daily needs. This allows some room for adding flavorings to these meals (described below), and healthy daily snacks, and drinks. If you are concerned about or experience weight gain, try to eat smaller portion sizes of these same meals.

In my opinion, what is more important for weight management than calorie counting is the food you consume. Several studies show that a healthy diet full of a variety of unprocessed animal and plant foods with recommended levels of macronutrients and micronutrients allows your metabolism, digestive system, and gut microbiota to perform as intended. It will provide you with the necessary energy to be active, keep you full longer so you don't overeat, support weight management, and promote overall good health.

In addition, limiting your diet's intake of added sugar, sodium, and saturated fat to no more than recommended levels helps support weight management and keeps your body from being negatively affected by unnaturally high levels of harmful additives.

The meals in this section are a good starting point for building such a diet.

Sources used for calories and weight description [231] [232]

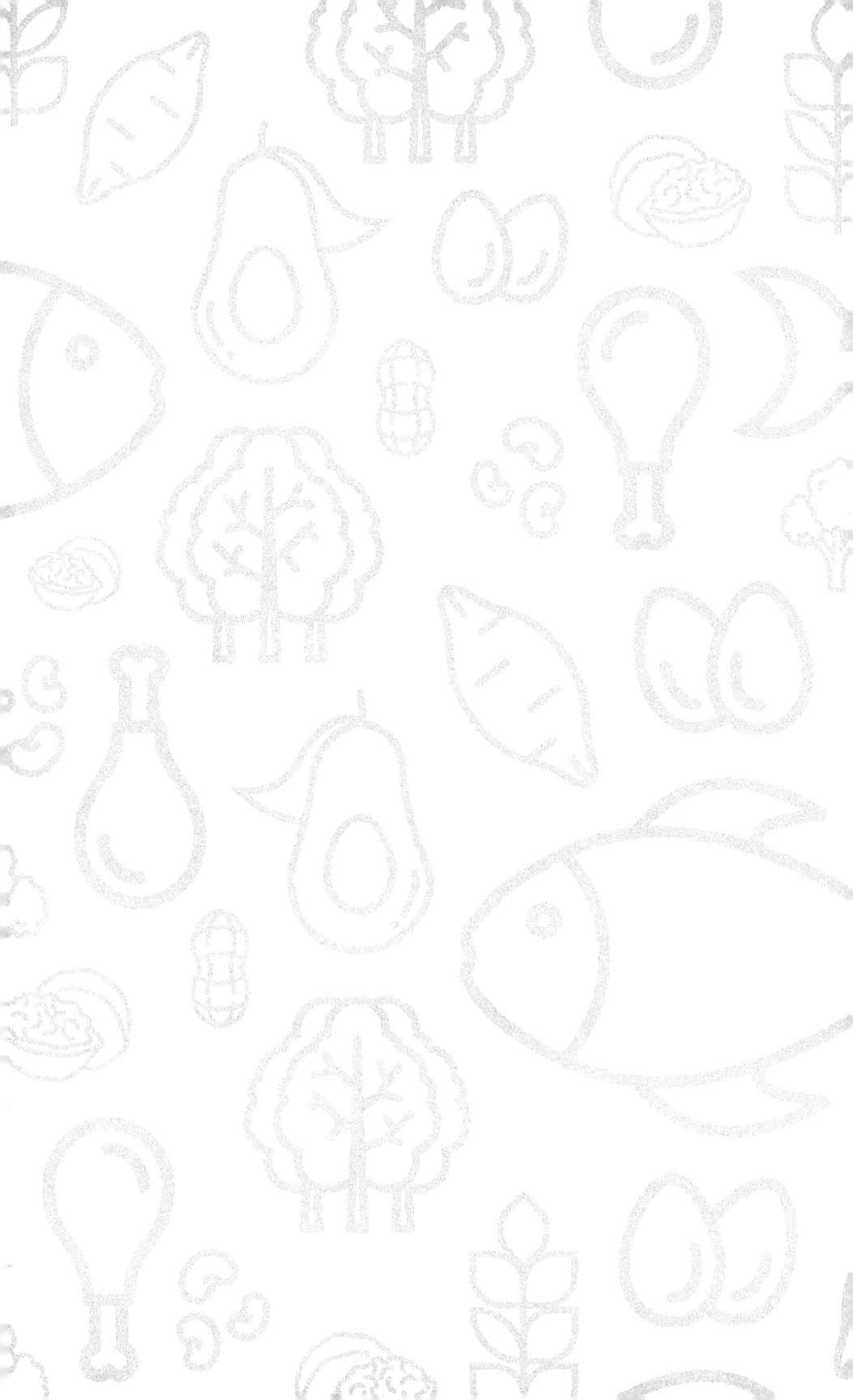

CHAPTER 17

How to Build Healthy Meals

I n the next chapter, I describe several very nutritious meals, made using the top 10, honorable mention, and other highly nutritious foods described in Section IV.

Before jumping in, I want to provide you with some general guidelines for building your own healthy meals. These include overall good meal habits, plus healthy strategies for selecting, preparing, and flavoring your foods. Lastly, I will describe a method for developing healthy meals that can really enhance nutrient levels. I call this my bowl strategy.

Good Meal Habits

Here are some healthy habits to consider for your daily and weekly meals:

- **Plan your meals in advance:** Buy foods and ingredients that support your planned meals, plus one to two healthy snacks. Choose snacks wisely. If you are like me, once you've bought a highly processed food (like ice cream) it's hard to make it an occasional snack (I usually consume it all within the week or less).

- **Use the nutrition facts labels when selecting foods:** Do so on all your store-bought foods to ensure you are making healthy choices.
- **Consume three meals every day:** If you skip meals, it will be difficult to meet daily nutrient recommended levels. Skipping meals will likely not help you lose weight. This strategy slows your metabolism and may cause you to overeat during other meals and make unhealthy food decisions.
- **Use portion control:** Large portions are usually fully consumed. If you have trouble with this, try reduced portions or use smaller plates.
- **Make as many meals at home as possible:** This will ensure you know your foods' ingredients and portion sizes, and you save lots of money!
- **Eat slowly and chew your food thoroughly:** This promotes feeling full and eating less. It also improves nutrient absorption.
- **Make this diet your routine:** We are creatures of habit and will follow these habits whether they're good or bad. Make them good!

Healthy Meal Development Strategies

To achieve a nutritious diet and limit unhealthy levels of added sugar, sodium, and saturated fat, consider implementing the following strategies.

Choose animal foods with healthy fat profiles: Fatty fish, poultry, and eggs are on my top 10 list, so I recommend these be regular choices. Shellfish are also a good addition to your meals. I recommend eating a variety of these animal foods weekly.

Dairy is another animal food you should consider. Studies show greek yogurt, kefir, and milk at typical serving sizes are healthy for us. There are some nutritional questions on whether lower fat options are better for us than full fat. More research is needed on this issue. So, for now select the dairy products at fat levels that suit your tastes.

As for red meat, I recommend consuming no more than one serving per week and choosing lean cuts or ground meats with 10% or less fat. I describe these cuts and healthy red meat strategies in Section IV. This approach is even more important for those who have cardiovascular health issues or high cholesterol.

Overall, one to four servings of animal-based foods per day for adults is a healthy approach. This leaves plenty of room for plant foods. In terms of serving sizes, I suggest limiting yourself to 6–8 ounces of meat daily. Note that meat sizes are sometimes referred to in terms of a deck of cards. 6–8 ounces is approximately two decks of cards.

For eggs, one to three per meal is healthy. As for dairy, recommendations for adults range up to three servings per day using typical portion sizes. If you are lactose intolerant, you may want to consider a plain, plant-based milk product as these often add calcium and other important nutrients that typically come from dairy. Be careful of the sugar content in plant-based milks.

With this approach to animal foods, your diet will provide you with healthy saturated fat levels and support you in reaching recommended daily levels of protein, unsaturated fats, several B vitamins, vitamins A and D, and choline. These animal foods will also help you meet the daily recommended mineral levels for magnesium, potassium, iron, calcium, and zinc.

Note that if you do have specific medical issues, you should consult with your physician or a dietician before changing your animal food diet.

Include a variety of plant-based foods in every meal: Americans don't eat enough plant foods daily. To have a healthy diet, we must consume these in much greater frequency. There are credible health and nutrition recommendations for consuming at least 30 different plant foods a week. Remember, we humans evolved by eating a diet full of a large variety of plant-based foods.

The most nutrient-dense plant foods include broccoli, kale, sweet potatoes (with skin), avocados, legumes, peanuts, tree nuts, 100% whole-grain bread, quinoa, and several different berries and seeds. Other great choices include spinach, asparagus, potatoes (with skin), carrots, onions, garlic, peppers, tomatoes, citrus fruits, bananas, apples, long-grain brown rice, corn, and oats.

I recommend you try to consume at least 5–10 plant-based foods per day. With coffee and tea counting towards this total, and using meal strategies like salads, smoothies, oatmeal, and whole-grain breakfast cereal, it is not difficult to get to this daily level. I average around 15–20 different plant foods per day without much difficulty. The meal examples described later will get you to this level, and I have specifically noted the number of plant foods in each meal.

This plant-based strategy will help you achieve healthy levels of carbohydrates; fiber; vitamins A, B9 (folate), C, E, and K, most priority minerals, and numerous phytonutrients and antioxidants. In addition, many plants support a diet's overall healthy fat profile.

Use healthy cooking methods: Overall, cooking helps to increase the absorption of nutrients. However, it can reduce some nutrients in plant-based foods, especially when boiling and poaching. These methods cause nutrients to leach out into their water. Generally, the best cooking methods for plant nutrient retention are steaming, microwaving, blanching, roasting, baking, and sautéing.

For animal-based foods, nutrients can also be lost when cooking, especially at high temperatures. These methods can also cause the formation of harmful chemicals. Try using low to medium heat cooking methods for these foods. Slow cooking, pressure cooking, and sous vide are great methods for retaining animal foods' nutrients. "Low and slow" can yield some tender, delicious meat dishes.

Put flavor into your meals without adding sugar and salt: There are several strategies for adding flavor to meals without unhealthy levels of salt and sugar. Many of these healthy flavor enhancers are included late in the cooking process to ensure you get their full flavors. Some of the best, and those that add important nutrients, are:

- **Herbs and spices:** These are a healthy way to add flavor and phytonutrients to your meals. Some examples:

  - Basil and oregano add flavor to tomato dishes.
  - Dill is great with fish.
  - Rosmary complements the taste of chicken and pork.
  - Cilantro is great with chilis and salsas.
  - Dried chili peppers add great heat to a dish.
  - Other popular spices include cumin, cinnamon, garlic powder, smoked paprika, nutmeg, and turmeric.

- **Citrus:** The juice and zest from lemons, limes, and oranges can add wonderful flavor. Some of the best combinations are:

  - Lemon with fish and chicken dishes.
  - Lime with chilis and guacamole.
  - The zest and juice from an orange to marinate meats overnight. This tenderizes red meats and adds great flavor.

- **Vinegar:** A splash of vinegar can add dynamic flavor to salad dressings, chicken dishes, and certain vegetables.

Try my bowl meal strategy: Lastly, you will notice as you review the meals below that there are a lot of bowl meals. By this, I mean pasta sauces, chilis, stir fries, oatmeal, soups, etc. I also include smoothies in this category, although those aren't typically eaten from a bowl.

Why do I use these meals so often? For a few reasons:

- They are simple to prepare, and extra amounts can be refrigerated or frozen for future meals.
- It's easy to incorporate numerous healthy animal-based and plant-based foods into these dishes.
- You can add nutritious foods that you may not care for as their taste typically gets lost in the overall dish's taste.
- As explained above, food nutrients are lost with certain cooking methods. Because these bowl meals maintain all their cooking liquid, any nutrients that leach out of the foods are still consumed.
- There is a multitude of delicious recipes for these types of dishes online and many are quick, cost-effective, and easy to prepare, often in under an hour.

Now, let's move on to the example meals. Enjoy!

Sources used for building healthy meals description: [233] [234] [235] [236] [237] [238] [239] [240]

CHAPTER 18

Nutritious Breakfasts

The next three chapters provide examples of daily breakfasts, lunches, and dinners that have very high levels of nutrition. For each meal, I provide a list of ingredients, serving sizes, calories, a nutrient summary, and certain dietary considerations. I have also included a table that summarizes each meal's various nutrient values, presented as a percentage of their daily recommendation.

As described earlier in the book, the nutrient content of foods and meals is greatly impacted by the exact food consumed, serving size, cooking ingredients, and cooking method. I used the USDA FoodData Central website "legacy foods" section for almost all of the foods listed in these meals. I calculated these foods' nutrients values based on typical U.S. serving sizes. There wasn't always a perfect food match in the FoodData Central database, but I believe I selected ones that well represent the foods listed in these meals and their overall nutrient values.

In these analyses, I have highlighted where nutrient levels are below moderate levels (<10% of DRI) or where saturated fat, sodium, or natural sugar levels are unusually high by bolding and underlining the nutrient. Remember, no food or meal is nutritionally perfect (although a few of these are pretty darn close).

At the end of this section, I provide the nutritional results of consuming these meals as your daily diet. I think you will be happy with these nutrient results!

Unless the meal has fatty fish or some shellfish, the omega-3 EPA/DHA content of a meal will be very low. Therefore, I do not address this in the meal Nutrient Summary or Dietary Considerations but rather recommend a strategy for this important nutrient in the last chapter of this section.

Lastly, the meal examples below are not recipes. They are the key foods to include in meals and do not include spices, sauces, and flavoring methods. You can get an almost infinite number of recipes online.

Finally, at current food prices nearly all of these meals cost less than $10 per serving with most in the $4–6 range. When costing more than $10 per serving, I have made recommendations to reduce the costs.

Oatmeal Bowl – 785 calories

Per-Serving Ingredients: Oatmeal (½ cup), walnuts or almonds (handful—30g), mixed berries (blueberries, blackberries, and raspberries—1 cup), peanut butter (2 ¼ tablespoons), whey or pea protein powder (normally 2 scoops), chia seeds (2 tablespoons). Totals 5–6 plant-based foods.

Nutrient Summary: Great breakfast with two top 10 and two honorable mention foods. Provides high levels of protein and fiber and moderate carbohydrates and natural sugar. Excellent fat profile with ratio of 5:1 unsaturated fats to saturated fats.

Contains high levels of most vitamins except A, B12, D, and choline. Plants don't have B12 and D, and most have low levels of choline. The meal has all priority minerals at high levels. Very low in sodium.

Dietary Considerations: To compensate for lower vitamin levels, consider tuna, Atlantic salmon, rainbow trout, eggs, and fortified whole milk for your day's other meals. These all have healthy levels of A, B12, D, and choline. Also, the plant foods sweet potatoes, carrots, red peppers, leafy greens, and kale are all high in A.

Relatively high caloric breakfast. If weight management is a concern, try smaller portions of each ingredient.

Oatmeal Bowl

Macronutrients	% of DRI	Vitamins	% of DRI	Minerals	% of DRI
Calories:	785 kJ / 31%	*A*	*1%*	Priority:	
Protein:	47 g / 47%	B1	34%	Magnesium	72%
Fats:		B2	32%	Potassium	27%
Saturated	7 g / 25%	B3	58%	Iron	*67% / 30%
Monounsaturated	17 g / 49%	B5	24%	Zinc	45%
Omega-6	14.5 g / 100%	B6	26%	Calcium	**29% / 36%
Omega-3 ALA	6 g / 429%	B9	24%	Sodium	1%
Omega-3 EPA/DHA	*0 g / 0%*	*B12*	*0%*	Others:	
Unsat/Saturated Ratio:	5:1 Excellent	C	32%	Phosphorus	80%
Total Carbohydrates:	55.5 g / 17%	*D*	*0%*	Copper	111%
Natural Sugar	16.5 g / 18%	E	57%	Manganese	169%
Fiber	21 g / 60%	K	22%	Selenium	39%
		Choline	12%		

Source: USDA Food Data Central
DRI Level Scale: Very high: 50%+, High: 20-49%, Moderate: 10-19%
*Men/Women   **Based on protein powder (pea/whey)
Potential Nutritional Gap/Risk

Eggs – 475 calories

Per-Serving Ingredients: Medium eggs (2), 100% whole-wheat toast (1 slice), medium avocado (½), medium tangerines (2). Totals 3 plant-based foods.

Nutrient Summary: Low-calorie breakfast with three top 10 foods. Moderate in protein and carbohydrates. High in fiber and natural sugar. Very good fat profile with a 3:1 ratio.

Excellent vitamin profile with high levels of all except D (moderate level). Contains all priority minerals at high levels. Sodium level is moderate. Note that I used a lower sodium 100% whole-wheat bread than the USDA FoodData Central product for this meal analysis (and those below). My reasoning is that almost all popular U.S. 100% whole-wheat bread brands were substantially lower. I used an average sodium level of these brands.

Dietary Considerations: To achieve higher levels of protein and vitamin D, you could add another egg. This raises the protein and vitamin D to high levels and only adds 75 calories.

Make sure to select 100% whole-wheat bread that is low in sodium and added sugar. Some products add high levels of these to improve taste.

Eggs

Macronutrients	% of DRI	Vitamins	% of DRI	Minerals	% of DRI
Calories:	475 kJ / 19%	A	27%	**Priority:**	
Protein:	21 g / 21%	B1	33%	Magnesium	25%
Fats:		B2	58%	Potassium	29%
Saturated	5 g / 18%	B3	28%	Iron	*45% / 20%
Monounsaturated	12 g / 35%	B5	64%	Zinc	28%
Omega-6	4 g / 28%	B6	45%	Calcium	20%
Omega-3 ALA	0.3 g / 23%	B9	38%	Sodium	14%
Omega-3 EPA/DHA	*0.04 g / 2%*	B12	37%	**Others:**	
Unsat/Saturated Ratio:	3:1 Very Good	C	58%	Phosphorus	53%
Total Carbohydrates:	49 g / 15%	D	12%	Copper	29%
Natural Sugar	20 g / 23%	E	28%	Manganese	62%
Fiber	10.5 g / 31%	K	27%	Selenium	80%
		Choline	69%		

Source: USDA Food Data Central

DRI Level Scale: Very high: 50%+, High: 20-49%, Moderate: 10-19%

*Men/Women

Potential Nutritional Gap/Risk

Greek Yogurt Bowl — 490 calories

Per-Serving Ingredients: Low fat plain greek yogurt (¾ cup), walnuts or almonds (handful—30g), mixed berries (1 cup), chia seeds (2 tablespoons). Totals 3 plant-based foods.

Nutrient Summary: Includes one top 10 and two honorable mention foods. High in protein and fiber, and moderate in carbohydrates and natural sugar. An excellent fat ratio of 6:1.

Very good vitamin profile with high levels of most vitamins. Moderate levels of B9 and choline, except A, B5, and D. It has all priority minerals at high levels. The sodium level is low.

Dietary Considerations: You can boost the B5, B9, and choline levels to high by adding a slice of whole-wheat bread with 2 tablespoons of peanut butter. This brings the calorie total up to 800 calories, which is not too high unless you have weight management concerns. An alternative is to have the peanut butter bread with your lunch.

For the day's other meals, consider increasing vitamin A levels by consuming sweet potatoes, carrots, red peppers, leafy greens, and kale. Eggs are also an option, as they are high in A and moderate in D.

Greek Yogurt Bowl

Macronutrients	% of DRI	Vitamins	% of DRI	Minerals	% of DRI
Calories:	490 kJ / 20%	_A_	_3%_	**Priority:**	
Protein:	28 g / 28%	B1	24%	Magnesium	52%
Fats:		B2	48%	Potassium	23%
Saturated	3.5 g / 13%	B3	26%	Iron	*46% / 21%
Monounsaturated	7.5 g / 21%	_B5_	_9%_	Zinc	34%
Omega-6	9 g / 64%	B6	21%	Calcium	42%
Omega-3 ALA	6 g / 429%	B9	18%	Sodium	4%
Omega-3 EPA/DHA	_0 g / 0%_	B12	49%	**Others:**	
Unsat/Saturated Ratio:	6:1 Excellent	C	32%	Phosphorus	84%
Total Carbohydrates:	38 g / 12%	_D_	_0%_	Copper	89%
Natural Sugar	16 g / 18%	E	34%	Manganese	110%
Fiber	17.5 g / 50%	K	22%	Selenium	57%
		Choline	11%		

Source: USDA Food Data Central
DRI Level Scale: Very high: 50%+, High: 20-49%, Moderate: 10-19%
*Men/Women
Potential Nutritional Gap/Risk

Orange Smoothie – 405 calories

Per-Serving Ingredients: Medium orange (1), raw carrots (1 ½ medium), walnuts or almonds (handful), raw spinach (1 cup), whey or pea protein powder (normally 2 scoops). Totals 4–5 plant-based foods.

Nutrient Summary: Includes one top 10 and three nutritious foods (orange, spinach, and carrot). High in protein, fiber, and natural sugar, and low in carbohydrates. Fat ratio is outstanding at 7.5:1.

Vitamin profile is very good with high levels of most and moderate levels of B3 and B5. Low in B12, D, and choline. Has all priority minerals at high levels, except zinc and iron (women) at moderate levels. Sodium level is very low, as is selenium.

Dietary Considerations: Adding 2 tablespoons of peanut butter would raise B3, B5, and zinc levels to high, and choline to a moderate level. This only increases the total calories to 625.

For other meals, consider eating healthy meats, eggs, and dairy, as these are all high in B12 and choline. Eggs and fortified milk (or plant-based milk) can also provide healthy levels of vitamin D.

Orange Smoothie

Macronutrients	% of DRI	Vitamins	% of DRI	Minerals	% of DRI
Calories:	405 kJ / 16%	A	72%	**Priority:**	
Protein:	33 g / 33%	B1	22%	Magnesium	31%
Fats:		B2	29%	Potassium	29%
Saturated	2 g / 7%	B3	12%	Iron	*27% / 12%
Monounsaturated	6.5 g / 18%	B5	13%	Zinc	13%
Omega-6	7.5 g / 53%	B6	24%	Calcium	**19% / 26%
Omega-3 ALA	1.5 g / 105%	B9	34%	Sodium	4%
Omega-3 EPA/DHA	*0 g / 0%*	*B12*	*0%*	**Others:**	
Unsat/Saturated Ratio:	7.5:1 Excellent	C	111%	Phosphorus	25%
Total Carbohydrates:	32 g / 10%	*D*	*0%*	Copper	59%
Natural Sugar	19.5 g / 22%	E	33%	Manganese	60%
Fiber	8.5 g / 24%	K	145%	*Selenium*	*4%*
		Choline	*8%*		

Source: USDA Food Data Central
DRI Level Scale: Very high: 50%+, High: 20-49%, Moderate: 10-19%
*Men/Women   **Based on protein powder (pea/whey)
Potential Nutritional Gap/Risk

Cereal/Shredded Wheat – 500 calories

Per-Serving Ingredients: Shredded 100% whole wheat (1 ⅓ cup), whole milk (fortified—1 cup), mixed berries (1 cup), ground flax seeds (2 tablespoons). Totals 3 plant-based foods.

Nutrient Summary: Includes one top 10 and two honorable mention foods. Provides moderate levels of protein, and high levels of fiber, carbohydrates, and natural sugar. It has a poor fat ratio of 1.5:1.

Vitamin profile is very good, with high levels of several and moderate amounts of A, B9, E, and choline. It has a great mineral profile with all priority minerals at high levels. Low in sodium.

Dietary Considerations: To supplement its nutrients, you could add a handful of almonds, raising protein, B9, and E to high levels. This also raises choline a little higher and improves the fat profile by adding healthy levels of monounsaturated and omega-6 fatty acids. It would add only 180 calories.

For your other meals, try eating sweet potatoes, carrots, red peppers, leafy greens, and kale to raise vitamin A levels.

The high sugar levels and poor fat ratio result from the milk. These are not major health concerns depending on your other meals that day. An alternative is to substitute low-sugar plant-based milk to improve the fat profile and lower the sugar. These are often fortified with A, B12, D, and calcium.

Make sure to select 100% whole grains for your cereal with low levels of added sugar and sodium.

Cereal/Shredded Wheat

Macronutrients	% of DRI	Vitamins	% of DRI	Minerals	% of DRI
Calories:	500 kJ / 20%	A	15%	Priority:	
Protein:	18 g / 18%	B1	31%	Magnesium	56%
Fats:		B2	43%	Potassium	29%
Saturated	5.5 g / 19%	B3	31%	Iron	*49% / 22%
Monounsaturated	*3 g / 9%*	B5	25%	Zinc	40%
Omega-6	2 g / 14%	B6	20%	Calcium	37%
Omega-3 ALA	3 g / 227%	B9	15%	Sodium	8%
Omega-3 EPA/DHA	*0 g / 0%*	B12	47%	Others:	
Unsat/Saturated Ratio:	*1.5:1 Poor*	C	31%	Phosphorus	81%
Total Carbohydrates:	82 g / 25%	D	22%	Copper	25%
Natural Sugar	22.5 g / 25%	E	14%	Manganese	54%
Fiber	18.5 g / 53%	K	24%	Selenium	61%
		Choline	13%		

Source: USDA Food Data Central
DRI Level Scale: Very high: 50%+, High: 20-49%, Moderate: 10-19%
*Men/Women

Potential Nutritional Gap/Risk

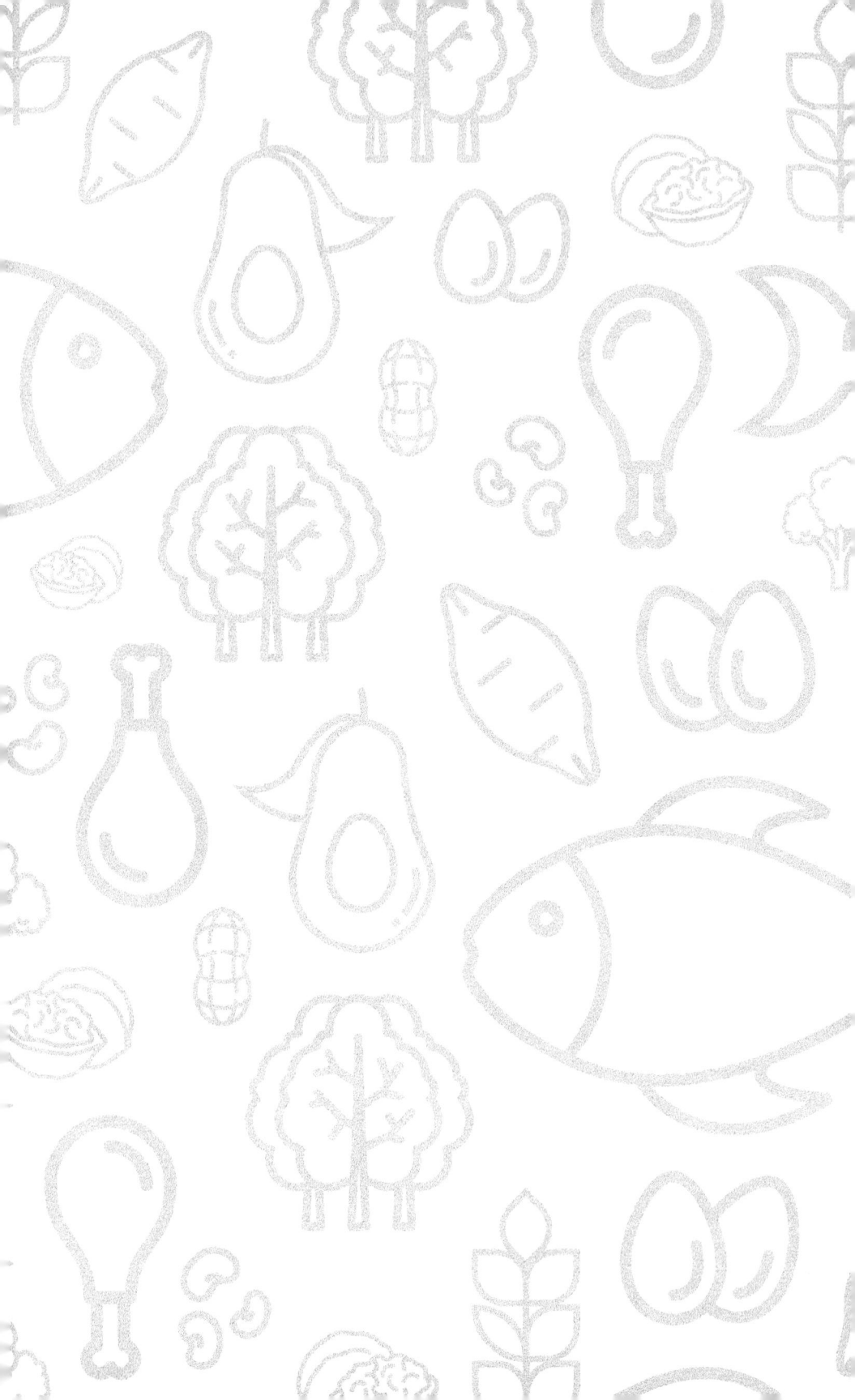

CHAPTER 19

Nutritious Lunches

Tuna Salad - 580 calories

Per-Serving Ingredients: Chunk light tuna fish (5-ounce can), hummus (4 tablespoons), medium avocado (1), raw chopped red sweet peppers (½ cup), celery (1 stalk), chopped romaine lettuce (1 cup). Totals 5 plant-based foods.

Nutrient Summary: This lunch uses two top 10 and one honorable mention foods. It is high in protein and fiber, and low in carbohydrates and natural sugar. Its fat ratio is excellent at 5:1.

Outstanding vitamin profile with high levels of all except choline. Great mineral profile with all priority minerals at high levels, except calcium at 10% of the DRI. Moderate in sodium.

Dietary Considerations: It's hard to beat this meal's nutrient profile. This would make a healthy dinner as well as a salad or sandwich. Two slices of low sodium 100% whole-wheat bread further enhances this meal's already excellent nutrient profile and takes calcium up to high levels. This increases the calorie total up to 830. If you have weight management concerns, use half an avocado.

Light or chunk light tuna, sometimes called skipjack, is healthy and has low levels of mercury. Also, many canned tuna products add salt, which raises the sodium levels. Try selecting one that has no salt added and make sure your canned tuna has healthy levels of vitamin D.

Tuna Salad

Macronutrients	% of DRI	Vitamins	% of DRI	Minerals	% of DRI
Calories:	580 kJ / 23%	A	44%	Priority:	
Protein:	45 g / 45%	B1	28%	Magnesium	41%
Fats:		B2	41%	Potassium	54%
Saturated	5 g / 18%	B3	152%	Iron	*67% / 30%
Monounsaturated	18 g / 52%	B5	60%	Zinc	32%
Omega-6	7.5 g / 52%	B6	96%	Calcium	10%
Omega-3 ALA	.7 g / 51%	B9	67%	Sodium	15%
Omega-3 EPA/DHA	0.4 g / 16%	B12	174%	Others:	
Unsat/Saturated Ratio:	5:1 Excellent	C	138%	Phosphorus	65%
Total Carbohydrates:	29 g / 9%	D	32%	Copper	42%
Natural Sugar	5.5 g / 6%	E	50%	Manganese	55%
Fiber	16.5 g / 47%	K	107%	Selenium	212%
		Choline	18%		

Source: USDA Food Data Central
DRI Level Scale: Very high: 50%+, High: 20-49%, Moderate: 10-19%
*Men/Women

Potential Nutritional Gap/Risk

Sliced Chicken Sandwich – 660 calories

Per-Serving Ingredients: Chicken breast (6 ounces, sliced), medium avocado (½), whole-wheat bread (2 slices), red tomato (2 slices). Totals 3 plant-based foods.

Nutrient Summary: Uses three top 10 foods. Provides high levels of protein and fiber, is moderate in carbohydrates and low in natural sugar. It has a very good fat profile ratio of 3.5:1.

Vitamin profile is very good, with most essential vitamins and choline at high levels. Exceptions are A and D at very low levels. Mineral profile is excellent, with all priority minerals at high levels.

Dietary Considerations: To supplement its nutrients, try adding 1 cup of romaine lettuce or half a baked sweet potato to this meal. Both will take the vitamin A up to high levels.

As mentioned above, use lower sodium (and calorie) 100% whole-wheat bread options.

Chicken Sandwich

Macronutrients	% of DRI	Vitamins	% of DRI	Minerals	% of DRI
Calories:	660 kJ / 26%	*A*	*4%*	Priority:	
Protein:	67 g / 67%	B1	50%	Magnesium	42%
Fats:		B2	39%	Potassium	38%
Saturated	4 g / 14%	B3	195%	Iron	*59% / 26%
Monounsaturated	10 g / 29%	B5	67%	Zinc	40%
Omega-6	3.5 g / 26%	B6	112%	Calcium	20%
Omega-3 ALA	.3 g / 20%	B9	29%	Sodium	17%
Omega-3 EPA/DHA	*0.1 g / 2%*	B12	24%	Others:	
Unsat/Saturated Ratio:	3.5:1 Very Good	C	16%	Phosphorus	93%
Total Carbohydrates:	51 g / 16%	*D*	*1%*	Copper	39%
Natural Sugar	6 g / 7%	E	33%	Manganese	115%
Fiber	11.5 g / 33%	K	26%	Selenium	133%
		Choline	38%		

Source: USDA Food Data Central
DRI Level Scale: Very high: 50%+, High: 20-49%, Moderate: 10-19%
*Men/Women
Potential Nutritional Gap/Risk

Apple Smoothie – 455 calories

Per-Serving Ingredients: Medium apple (½), medium kiwi (1), avocado (½), raw spinach (1 cup), whey or pea protein powder (normally 2 scoops), chia seeds (2 tablespoons). Totals 5–6 plant-based foods.

Nutrient Summary: Includes one top 10 and two honorable mention foods. It has high levels of protein and fiber and is moderate in carbohydrates. Slightly high in natural sugar, and I used only half an apple to keep it from being higher. It has an excellent fat ratio of 5:1.

Vitamin profile is very good with several at high levels, except B12, D, and choline at low levels. Its mineral profile is excellent with all priority minerals at high levels (zinc at 19%). It has very low levels of sodium.

Dietary Considerations: Adding 1 cup of milk or ¾ cup of plain greek yogurt would raise the B12 level to high and choline to moderate. If fortified, the milk would also add A and D. These dairy foods only add 100–150 calories. To keep the meal vegan, consider plant-based milk, as several are fortified with A, B12, D, and calcium.

Apple Smoothie

Macronutrients	% of DRI	Vitamins	% of DRI	Minerals	% of DRI
Calories:	455 kJ / 18%	A	19%	Priority:	
Protein:	33 g / 33%	B1	22%	Magnesium	40%
Fats:		B2	20%	Potassium	35%
Saturated	3 g / 11%	B3	27%	Iron	*45% / 20%
Monounsaturated	8 g / 23%	B5	25%	Zinc	19%
Omega-6	3 g / 20%	B6	26%	Calcium	**25% / 32%
Omega-3 ALA	4.5 g / 329%	B9	38%	Sodium	2%
Omega-3 EPA/DHA	_0 g / 0%_	_B12_	_0%_	Others:	
Unsat/Saturated Ratio:	5:1 Excellent	C	114%	Phosphorus	42%
Total Carbohydrates:	44 g / 14%	_D_	_0%_	Copper	45%
Natural Sugar	18.5 g / 21%	E	24%	Manganese	55%
Fiber	18.5 g / 53%	K	185%	Selenium	34%
		Choline	_5%_		

Source: USDA Food Data Central
DRI Level Scale: Very high: 50%+, High: 20-49%, Moderate: 10-19%
*Men/Women   **Based on protein powder (pea/whey)

Potential Nutritional Gap/Risk

Peanut Butter Sandwich – 560 calories

Per-Serving Ingredients: Peanut butter (2 ¼ tablespoons)**,** 100% whole-wheat bread (2 slices), banana (½), tangerine (1). Totals 4 plant-based foods.

Nutrient Summary: Uses two top 10 foods. It is high in protein, fiber, carbohydrates, and natural sugar. With its fiber content, the high natural sugar should not be a major health concern. This sandwich has a very good fat ratio of 3.5:1.

Vitamin profile is good, with most essentials at high levels. The exceptions are A, B12, D, and K, which are at low levels. Its mineral profile is excellent with all priority minerals at high levels. It has moderate levels of sodium.

Dietary Considerations: Adding a glass of fortified milk (1 cup) or fortified plant-based milk increases vitamins A, B12, and D to high levels. Full fat milk would lower the fat ratio to 2:1, but this level is still healthy. These foods only add 200 calories to the meal.

For your other meals, try to consume foods with healthy levels of vitamin K. These include fatty fish, eggs, chicken, nuts, peanuts, avocados, several berries, and kiwi.

Try selecting peanut butter that uses all natural peanut ingredients and is low in sodium, with no added sugar. There are several peanut butter product options that fit this description.

Peanut Butter Sandwich

Macronutrients	% of DRI	Vitamins	% of DRI	Minerals	% of DRI
Calories:	560 kJ / 22%	_A_	_3%_	**Priority:**	
Protein:	22 g / 22%	B1	44%	Magnesium	45%
Fats:		B2	25%	Potassium	26%
Saturated	4.5 g / 17%	B3	66%	Iron	*42% / 19%
Monounsaturated	10.5 g / 30%	B5	28%	Zinc	29%
Omega-6	6 g / 42%	B6	48%	Calcium	21%
Omega-3 ALA	.2 g / 13%	B9	24%	Sodium	9%
Omega-3 EPA/DHA	_0 g / 0%_	_B12_	_0%_	**Others:**	
Unsat/Saturated Ratio:	3.5:1 Very Good	C	30%	Phosphorus	52%
Total Carbohydrates:	72.5 g / 22%	_D_	_0%_	Copper	51%
Natural Sugar	22 g / 25%	E	42%	Manganese	144%
Fiber	10.5 g / 30%	_K_	_8%_	Selenium	51%
		Choline	13%		

Source: USDA Food Data Central
DRI Level Scale: Very high: 50%+, High: 20-49%, Moderate: 10-19%
*Men/Women

Potential Nutritional Gap/Risk

Vegetarian Salad – 770 calories

Per-Serving Ingredients: Edamame (½ cup), sweet red peppers (½ cup), chickpeas (⅔ cup), cashews (handful), chopped butter lettuce (1 cup), olive oil (2 tablespoons to make a dressing). Totals 6 plant-based foods.

Nutrient Summary: Includes three top 10 foods (edamame, chickpeas, and cashews). It is high in protein and fiber, and moderate in carbohydrates and natural sugar.

It has an excellent fat ratio of 5:1. The relatively high saturated fat level comes from the olive oil and cashews. With very high levels of unsaturated fats and a healthy fat profile, the saturated fat should not be a health concern.

The vitamin profile is very good, with most essentials at high to very high levels, except B3 at moderate levels, and B12 and D at low levels. Its mineral profile is excellent with all priority minerals at high levels, except calcium at moderate levels. It is low in sodium.

Dietary Considerations: If concerned about the B3 and B12 levels, you could add 6 ounces of chicken to get these to high levels. This adds 280 calories which totals over 1,000 calories. This is a little high for a lunch for some people, but it is an incredibly healthy meal. It could be used as a dinner as well.

Vegetarian Salad

Macronutrients	% of DRI	Vitamins	% of DRI	Minerals	% of DRI
Calories:	770 kJ / 31%	A	31%	Priority:	
Protein:	29 g / 29%	B1	35%	Magnesium	60%
Fats:		B2	29%	Potassium	42%
Saturated	8 g / 28%	B3	17%	Iron	*107% / 47%
Monounsaturated	30 g / 86%	B5	26%	Zinc	51%
Omega-6	10 g / 65%	B6	60%	Calcium	16%
Omega-3 ALA	0.8 g / 62%	B9	126%	Sodium	8%
Omega-3 EPA/DHA	*0 g / 0%*	*B12*	*0%*	Others:	
Unsat/Saturated Ratio:	5:1 Excellent	C	128%	Phosphorus	79%
Total Carbohydrates:	53 g / 16%	*D*	*0%*	Copper	144%
Natural Sugar	13 g / 14%	E	42%	Manganese	108%
Fiber	16.5 g / 48%	K	110%	Selenium	17%
		Choline	28%		

Source: USDA Food Data Central
DRI Level Scale: Very high: 50%+, High: 20-49%, Moderate: 10-19%
*Men/Women

Potential Nutritional Gap/Risk

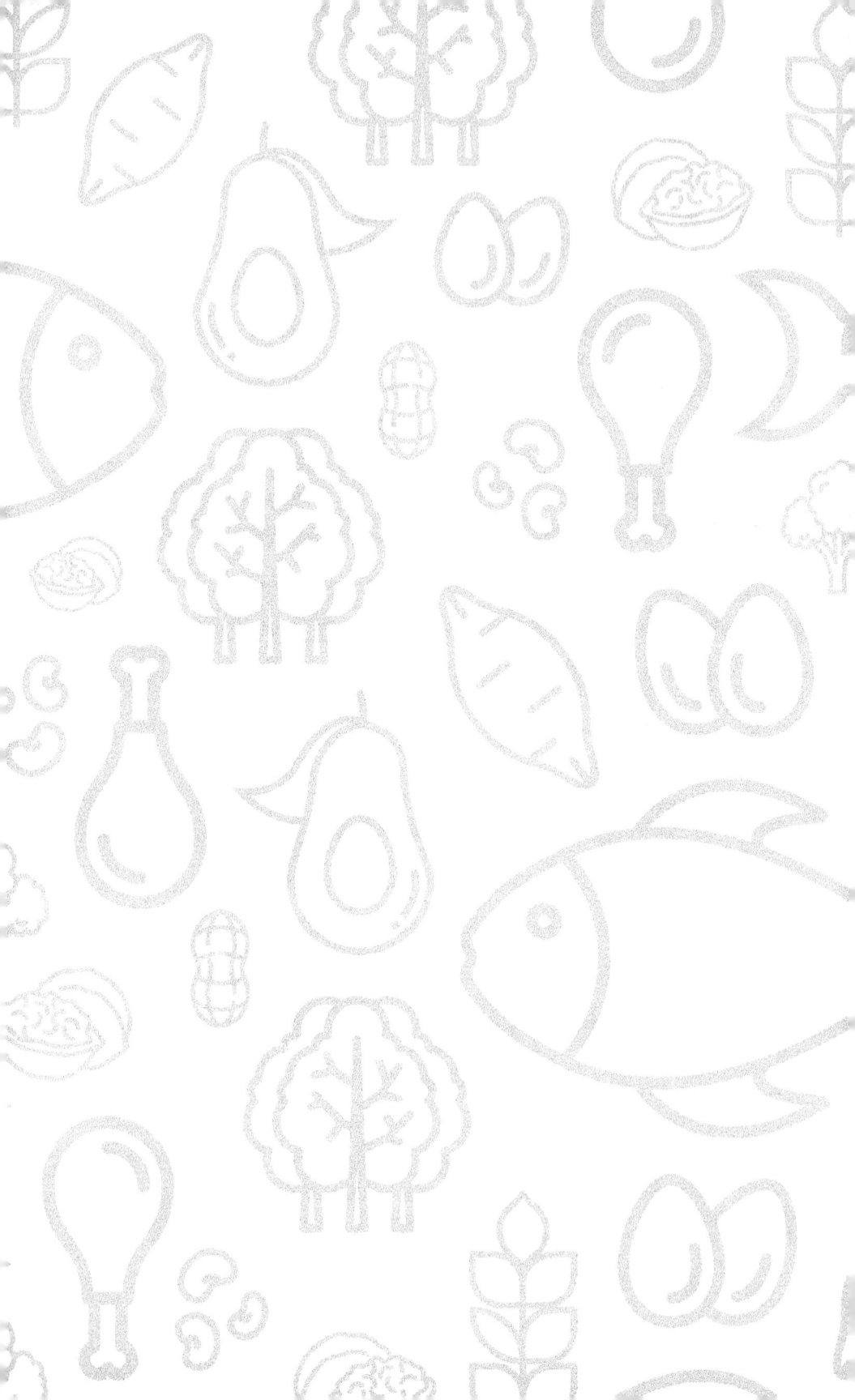

CHAPTER 20

Nutritious Dinners

Grilled Salmon – 800 calories

Per Serving Ingredients: Atlantic Salmon fillet (6 ounces), sauteed broccoli (1 cup), baked potato (medium), olive oil (2 tablespoons) to cook the fish and side dishes. Totals 3 plant-based foods.

Nutrient Summary: Includes two top 10 foods. Provides high levels of protein and fiber with low levels of carbohydrates and natural sugar. Somewhat high in saturated fat, but with an excellent fat ratio of 4.5:1.

Contains all essential vitamins at high levels. It has all priority minerals at high to very high levels, except calcium at moderate. Its sodium level is moderate.

Dietary Considerations: None. This is a nearly perfect nutritional meal. If the salmon fillet is too costly, canned salmon is a much cheaper alternative to fresh. Some canned salmon are high in calcium. Make sure your canned salmon does not have added salt.

Grilled Salmon

Macronutrients	% of DRI	Vitamins	% of DRI	Minerals	% of DRI
Calories:	800 kJ / 32%	A	29%	Priority:	
Protein:	45 g / 45%	B1	68%	Magnesium	36%
Fats:		B2	41%	Potassium	67%
Saturated	8 g / 29%	B3	113%	Iron	*45% / 20%
Monounsaturated	27 g / 77%	B5	82%	Zinc	20%
Omega-6	4 g / 27%	B6	148%	Calcium	11%
Omega-3 ALA	.6 g / 44%	B9	67%	Sodium	12%
Omega-3 EPA/DHA	3.7 g / 146%	B12	202%	Others:	
Unsat/Saturated Ratio:	4.5:1 Excellent	C	145%	Phosphorus	93%
Total Carbohydrates:	47 g / 14%	D	148%	Copper	42%
Natural Sugar	4 g / 5%	E	54%	Manganese	34%
Fiber	9 g / 25%	K	220%	Selenium	134%
		Choline	50%		

Source: USDA Food Data Central
DRI Level Scale: Very high: 50%+, High: 20-49%, Moderate: 10-19%
*Men/Women

Potential Nutritional Gap/Risk

Chicken, Shrimp, or Tofu Stir Fry—
670–730 calories

Per Serving Ingredients: Chicken breast (6 ounces) or jumbo shrimp (6 ounces—about 9 shrimp) or tofu (5.25 ounces), quinoa (¾ cup), chopped red sweet peppers (½ cup), chopped portobello mushrooms (½ cup), chopped broccoli (½ cup), chopped carrots (1/6 cup), chopped onions (1/6 cup), minced garlic (1 clove), 1 tablespoon of olive oil for cooking. Totals 8–9 plant-based foods.

I added ¼ cup of peanuts to the shrimp and tofu versions to get the protein to high levels.

Nutrient Summary: Nutrient levels vary based on the protein used but overall, all three versions are very similar. These stir fry meals use two to three top 10 foods (shrimp is not one) and add several other nutritious foods.

All three are high in protein and fiber, and moderate in carbohydrates and natural sugar. They have moderate to high levels of saturated fat, but excellent fat ratios of 4–5:1.

All versions have excellent vitamin profiles with high levels of all essentials except D. The tofu version is also low in B12. They contain all priority minerals at high levels, except calcium, for which the chicken and shrimp versions are moderate (tofu version is high). Sodium levels are low, except for the shrimp version. It is naturally high in sodium like some other shellfish.

Dietary Considerations: Not much to add as these are highly nutritious meals. Try not to add sauces to your stir fry that are high in sodium, sugar, or saturated fat.

Chicken Stir Fry+

Macronutrients	% of DRI	Vitamins	% of DRI	Minerals	% of DRI
Calories:	670 kJ / 27%	A	45%	Priority:	
Protein:	63 g / 63%	B1	38%	Magnesium	49%
Fats:		B2	50%	Potassium	45%
Saturated	4 g / 15%	B3	184%	Iron	*66% / 29%
Monounsaturated	13 g / 38%	B5	61%	Zinc	43%
Omega-6	4 g / 28%	B6	136%	Calcium	11%
Omega-3 ALA	0.4 g / 30%	B9	50%	Sodium	13%
Omega-3 EPA/DHA	*0.1 g / 3%*	B12	27%	Others:	
Unsat/Saturated Ratio:	4.5:1 Excellent	C	141%	Phosphorus	110%
Total Carbohydrates:	50 g / 15%	*D*	*2%*	Copper	70%
Natural Sugar	8 g / 9%	E	37%	Manganese	69%
Fiber	10 g / 28%	K	116%	Selenium	141%
		Choline	48%		

Source: USDA Food Data Central

DRI Level Scale: Very high: 50%+, High: 20-49%, Moderate: 10-19%

*Men/Women   + Includes only chicken version as all versions similar nutritionally

Potential Nutritional Gap/Risk

Pork Tenderloin—490 calories

Per Serving Ingredients: Pork tenderloin (6 ounces, lean), chopped asparagus (½ cup), black beans (⅔ cup), chopped green bell peppers (⅓ cup), chopped onions (1/6 cup), diced tomatoes (¼ cup), 1 tablespoon olive oil. The beans, peppers, onions, and tomatoes can be used to make a fresh black bean salad or cooked to develop one of several online dishes. Totals 6 plant-based foods.

Nutrient Summary: Uses one top 10 food. High in protein and fiber and low in carbohydrates and natural sugar. It is moderate in saturated fat. While the pork has a poor fat profile, the healthy fat profile of the other foods more than offsets this and results in a meal with an excellent fat ratio of 4:1.

Vitamin profile is high in all essentials, except A and D at low levels. All priority minerals are at high levels, except calcium. Sodium levels are high as a result of the pork product used by the USDA FoodData Central. Pork is naturally low in sodium, so try to use unprocessed meat for this meal.

Dietary Considerations: If you substitute 1 cup of cooked broccoli for the asparagus, the A and calcium levels go up to high and moderate, respectively.

Pork Tenderloin

Macronutrients	% of DRI	Vitamins	% of DRI	Minerals	% of DRI
Calories:	490 kJ / 20%	_A_	_6%_	Priority:	
Protein:	47 g / 47%	B1	152%	Magnesium	38%
Fats:		B2	67%	Potassium	57%
Saturated	3 g / 12%	B3	86%	Iron	*61% / 27%
Monounsaturated	11.5 g / 33%	B5	40%	Zinc	48%
Omega-6	2 g / 14%	B6	128%	_Calcium_	_7%_
Omega-3 ALA	0.3 g / 19%	B9	72%	Sodium	29%
Omega-3 EPA/DHA	_0 g / 0%_	B12	37%	Others:	
Unsat/Saturated Ratio:	4:1 Excellent	C	24%	Phosphorus	102%
Total Carbohydrates:	35 g / 11%	_D_	_2%_	Copper	68%
Natural Sugar	5.5 g / 6%	E	31%	Manganese	37%
Fiber	12 g / 34%	K	61%	Selenium	124%
		Choline	40%		

Source: USDA Food Data Central
DRI Level Scale: Very high: 50%+, High: 20-49%, Moderate: 10-19%
*Men/Women
Potential Nutritional Gap/Risk

Soybean, Chicken, or Beef Chili—685–875 calories

Per Serving Ingredients: Chicken breast (6 ounces), ground beef (93%/7% lean meat to fat–6 ounces), or soybeans (⅔ cup). In addition, canned stewed tomatoes (½ cup), black beans (½ cup), white beans (½ cup), chopped red sweet peppers (¼ cup), chopped onions (1/6 cup), minced garlic clove (1), tablespoon of olive oil (1) and medium avocado (½—put slices on top of chili). This totals 8–9 plant-based foods.

Nutrient Summary: Uses three to four top 10 foods. As with the stir fry, the specific nutrient levels depend on the protein source. However, all three versions are high in protein and fiber, and moderate in carbohydrates and natural sugar. The beef version is high in saturated fat but has a good fat ratio of 2.5:1. The chicken and soybean versions' fat ratios are excellent, at 4.5–5.5:1.

All have excellent vitamin profiles with high levels of essentials, except A (9-11%) and no D. The soybean version is low in B12. All versions have priority minerals at high levels, except calcium at moderate (soybean version at high levels). All three options are particularly helpful in meeting daily iron requirements for women.

Sodium levels are moderate to high. However, this can be reduced by selecting lower sodium versions of stewed tomatoes and canned beans than the ones used by the USDA database. There are a lot of low sodium products for these canned vegetables.

Dietary Considerations: Other vegetables to consider for your chili are hot peppers, small broccoli florets (or broccoli rice), spinach, or carrots. These would increase the vitamin A levels without adding any unhealthy levels of other nutrients. To increase the B12 in the soybean version, you could add ¼ cup of shredded cheese. This amount would maintain the fat ratio and sodium at healthy levels.

Soybean Chili+

Macronutrients	% of DRI	Vitamins	% of DRI	Minerals	% of DRI
Calories:	685 kJ / 27%	*A*	*9%*	Priority:	
Protein:	36 g / 36%	B1	51%	Magnesium	65%
Fats:		B2	47%	Potassium	66%
Saturated	5 g / 18%	B3	24%	Iron	*151% / 67%
Monounsaturated	19.5 g / 56%	B5	39%	Zinc	40%
Omega-6	7.5 g / 51%	B6	63%	Calcium	26%
Omega-3 ALA	1 g / 70%	B9	79%	Sodium	13%
Omega-3 EPA/DHA	*0 g / 0%*	*B12*	*2%*	Others:	
Unsat/Saturated Ratio:	5.5:1 Excellent	C	85%	Phosphorus	76%
Total Carbohydrates:	67 g / 21%	*D*	*0%*	Copper	109%
Natural Sugar	12 g / 13%	E	46%	Manganese	98%
Fiber	25 g / 71%	K	48%	Selenium	21%
		Choline	27%		

Source: USDA Food Data Central

DRI Level Scale: Very high: 50%+, High: 20-49%, Moderate: 10-19%

*Men/Women   +Includes only the soybean version as all versions similar nutritionally

Potential Nutritional Gap/Risk

Beef Bolognaise—835 calories

Per Serving Ingredients: Ground beef (6 ounces, 10% fat), red pasta sauce (1 cup), raw onions (½ cup), medium carrot (½), celery (½ stalk), garlic clove (1), egg noodles (handful—2 oz. or 56g is a typical serving size), and olive oil (1 tablespoon) to cook the vegetables and beef. Totals 7 plant-based foods.

🔍 DYK

Bolognaise purists will likely point out that there is no pork, milk, or wine in this meal. These items tend to add substantial amounts of saturated fat and calories, and if included would not make my nutritious meal list. It may be more accurate to describe this as a meat pasta sauce, but it is still delicious! There are many recipes for similar sauces online.

Nutrient Summary: This meal has no top 10 or honorable mention foods and is high in saturated fat. Nonetheless, by pairing several nutritious foods with the lean ground beef, this is still a recommended meal.

This meal provides high levels of protein, fiber, and carbohydrates, and is moderate in natural sugar. While it is high in saturated fat, the meal has a good fat ratio of 2:1. The olive oil, canned sauce, onion, garlic, and carrots all have fat ratios of over 3:1, which brings up the levels of unsaturated fats and improves the meal's overall ratio.

It contains all essential vitamins at high levels, except D, and has all priority minerals at high levels, except calcium (moderate). The sodium level is moderate.

Dietary Considerations: With its high saturated fat levels, this is a meal I would not recommend eating more than once a week. Using whole-wheat pasta, instead of the egg pasta, would further improve the fat profile. Also, I personally use an egg pasta that has no saturated fat and has a better fat profile than the one used by the USDA database.

Make sure to select a pasta sauce that is low in sodium and added sugar.

Beef Bolognaise

Macronutrients	% of DRI	Vitamins	% of DRI	Minerals	% of DRI
Calories:	835 kJ / 33%	A	36%	**Priority:**	
Protein:	58 g / 58%	B1	27%	Magnesium	35%
Fats:		B2	49%	Potassium	60%
Saturated	_10.5 g / 38%_	B3	92%	Iron	*108% / 48%
Monounsaturated	19.5 g / 56%	B5	55%	Zinc	128%
Omega-6	3 g / 21%	B6	106%	Calcium	13%
Omega-3 ALA	0.2 g / 18%	B9	20%	Sodium	13%
Omega-3 EPA/DHA	_0 g / 0%_	B12	190%	**Others:**	
Unsat/Saturated Ratio:	2:1 Good	C	29%	Phosphorus	87%
Total Carbohydrates:	70 g / 21%	_D_	_1%_	Copper	80%
Natural Sugar	17 g / 18%	E	43%	Manganese	54%
Fiber	8.5 g / 24%	K	26%	Selenium	152%
		Choline	46%		

Source: USDA Food Data Central
DRI Level Scale: Very high: 50%+, High: 20-49%, Moderate: 10-19%
*Men/Women
Potential Nutritional Gap/Risk

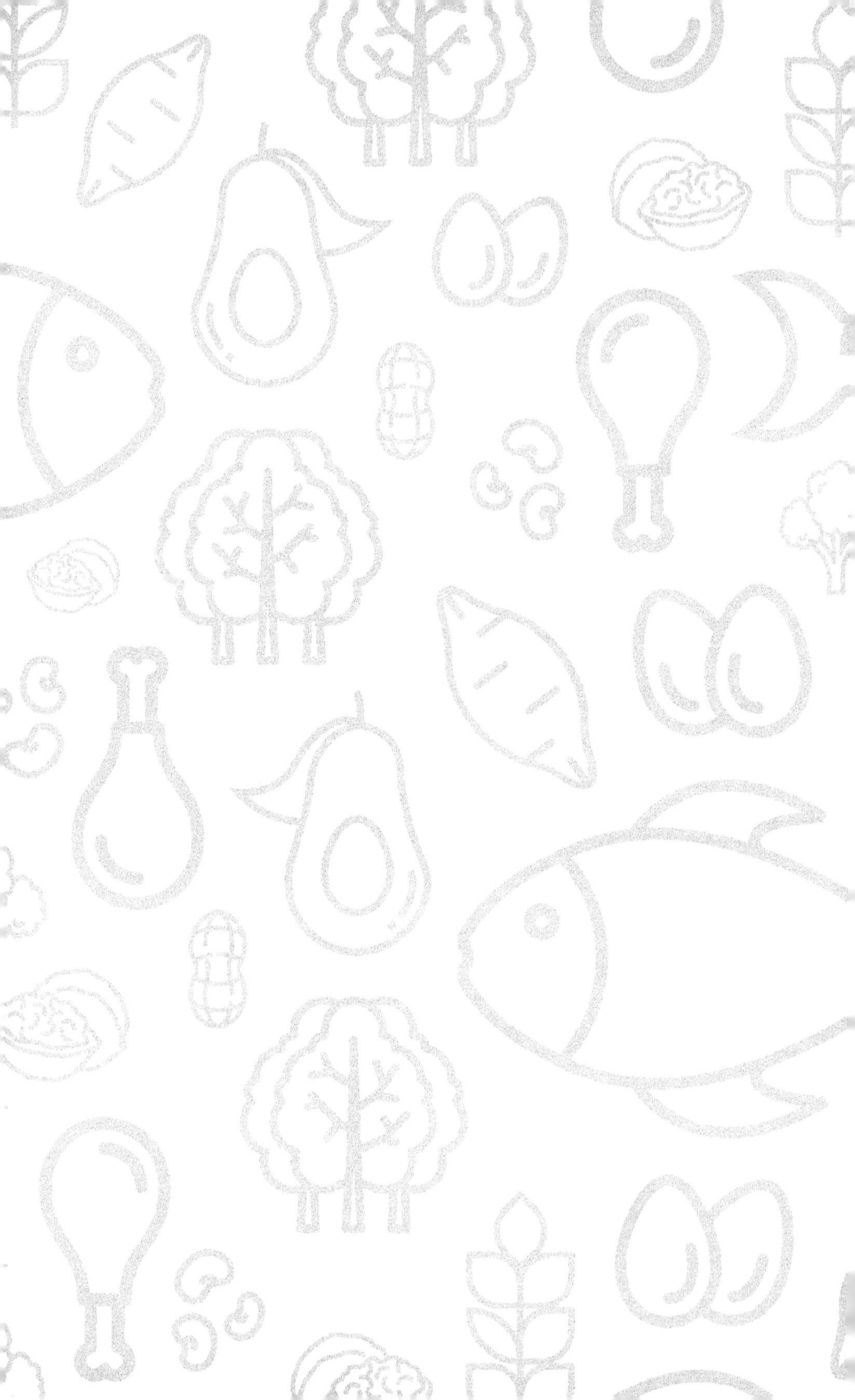

CHAPTER 21

Do the Example Meals Provide Absolute Nutrition?

I f you regularly consume nutrient-dense meals like those described in this section, you will achieve very close to full nutrition.

How do I know this? Because I added up the nutrient levels for all 15 meals in the last three chapters (actually, 19 with different stir fry and chili options), calculated a meal average for each nutrient and then multiplied this by three (for three meals a day). This provides a daily average for all nutrient levels if you were to consume only these meals.

According to the results, 22 of the total 32 macro and micro-nutrients measured came in above 100% of their DRIs. This includes protein, nearly all unsaturated fats, fiber, all B vitamins, vitamins C, E, and K, and nearly all minerals (priority and others). These meals also averaged 14 ½ plant foods daily. Not bad!

Many of these nutrients that reached their daily recommended levels are some of the ones that most Americans struggle to get. Also, the daily average ratio of unsaturated to saturated fat is an excellent 4:1. This means these meals are an outstanding strategy to support your cardiovascular health.

Lastly, the average calorie count is 1,850, or 75% of the 2,500 daily benchmark. This makes sense, because these meals do not include drinks, snacks, or additives for flavoring and cooking (e.g., sauces, oils, etc.). If you select healthy drinks, snacks, and flavoring, you will enhance the daily nutrient values without adding a great deal of calories.

Here is a summary of the nutrients where these meals fell a little short of the daily recommended levels. Note that under certain conditions I recommend you consider a nutrient supplement. Some supplements can interact poorly with certain medications, so please discuss this with your physician if you are on medication(s) or have a significant health condition.

The Good

Three of the nutrients not meeting the daily recommendations were **saturated fat** (59% of DRI), **natural sugar** (46%), and **sodium** (34%). This is an excellent outcome from a health perspective and allows some flexibility with meal flavoring.

The Bad (But Not *So* Bad)

Four of the remaining seven nutrients achieved over 70% of their daily recommendations. These are described below:

Vitamin A reached 71% of its DRI. This shortfall can be addressed by adding foods such as sweet potatoes, carrots, red peppers, leafy greens, and kale into your regular diet. These are all low-calorie additions, at 100 calories or less per typical serving. Put them in a smoothy or another bowl meal if you don't like their taste.

Choline came in at 87% of its DRI. Very close. This is likely the result of several vegetarian dishes being included in the list of meals. If you regularly consume a variety of animal-based foods (in addition to dairy), you should not worry about getting adequate choline. If you are vegan, discuss a supplement with your doctor or a dietician. The best plant foods for choline are soy products, peanuts, and some legumes, but at typical serving sizes these are all under 15% of the DRI.

Calcium reached 68% of its DRI. If you are not vegan or lactose intolerant, try consuming one to three servings of dairy per day to get adequate amounts. Plain greek yogurt and kefir are great choices. Whey protein powder also has 5–15% of the calcium DRI, depending on the brand.

If you don't consume dairy, try regularly eating kale, certain canned fatty fish, 100% whole-wheat bread, tofu, and chia seeds. These all have 15–25% of the DRI at typical serving sizes.

If you are vegan, try the plant foods listed above. In addition, many plant-based milks are fortified with calcium and are a good option to get this important nutrient. You can also consider a calcium supplement. Please do not exceed the UL as this can cause significant health issues and discuss supplements with a medical professional first.

Iron is the other mineral that fell just short of its DRI, but only for women at 87%. Female requirements for iron up to age 50 are almost 2.5 times that of males, so this is not surprising.

The best meals for women to get iron are the vegetarian salad (47% of DRI), bolognaise (49%), all chili meals (50–70%), and the vegetable stir fry (40%). Regularly consuming these or similar meals will help you get adequate iron. Also, individual foods with healthy levels of iron include oysters, sardines, beef, soybeans, legumes, game meats, tuna fish, eggs, 100% whole-wheat bread, quinoa, baked potato, tomato sauce, chia seeds, and spinach.

If you are considering an iron supplement, stay at or under the UL. It is best to discuss this supplement with your physician before starting.

The Ugly

Two of the remaining three nutrients are omega-3 EPA/DHA and vitamin D. These came in at 34% and 44% of their daily recommendations, respectively.

Omega-3 EPA/DHA is very difficult to get at recommended levels, as fatty fish is its main dietary source. If you are not a fish fan, I recommend you consider a supplement to get your totals up to 2–3 grams daily. Even if you do consume fatty fish twice a week, you are likely not reaching this level consistently. On the days I am not eating fatty fish, I take an omega-3 EPA/DHA supplement for this very reason. Please consider discussing this with your physician.

As for **vitamin D**, other than fatty fish, you can get healthy amounts from eggs and fortified milk. You also have an additional option to get this critical nutrient: sunlight on your skin for approximately 20 minutes is believed to provide adequate daily amounts. If you don't enjoy fatty fish or like to go outside, then you should strongly consider a supplement. Also, during the winter months with less sunlight and skin exposure to the sun you may also want to consider a supplement. Please do not take one at levels above the UL.

The Confusing

The meals' **carbohydrate** daily average is well below the FNB DRI of 45–65% daily calories. In fact, it's approximately 50% of the lower end. As I described in Section II, after looking at unprocessed plant-based foods considered high in carbs (e.g., potatoes, whole-wheat bread, quinoa, pasta, etc.) I found that they all have 15% or less of the DRI at typical serving sizes.

Given this, it is virtually impossible to reach the FNB recommended carbohydrate range by eating a well-balanced diet full of these unprocessed, complex carbohydrate foods. The only foods that would get you close to the recommended carbohydrate range are all highly processed, like pretzels, doughnuts, soft drinks, and bagels.

So, what do you do about the carb DRI? My recommendation is to ignore the FNB range and focus your diet on unprocessed plant foods. The average of the meals above provides close to 15 plant foods daily. Attaining this level provides you with healthy levels of complex carbohydrates, fiber, several important vitamins, most priority minerals, and numerous phytonutrients high in antioxidants. Many plants also help support a diet's healthy fat profile. Almost all credible health and nutrition sources recommend consuming whole, unprocessed plant foods for healthy carbohydrates. This is the strategy I use with carbohydrates and I have plenty of energy for my active lifestyle.

SECTION V KEY TAKEAWAYS

- **Establish nutritional goals.** If you define your goal as achieving absolute nutrition and limiting added sugar, sodium, and saturated fats, you are more likely to build a healthy diet. Focus more on selecting highly nutritious foods and meals than calorie counting.

- **Quit trying to be perfect.** Dietary perfection will lead to disappointment and likely quitting your plan. Try to stick to your healthy foods and meals at least five days a week. On off days, you can still follow some healthy food practices described in this section.

- **Develop good meal habits.** Plan your meals in advance, don't skip meals, limit the size of your food portions, and make meals at home when possible.

- **Use good meal development strategies:**

  - Choose animal foods with good fat profiles. Regularly consume unprocessed fatty fish, chicken, and eggs. All have fat ratios of at least twice as much unsaturated fat as saturated fat. Two to three servings of dairy per day is also healthy. Limit red meat to once a week. Use the food strategies described in this section and Section IV.

  - Get plenty of plant foods in your diet. Target daily consumption of at least five to ten unprocessed plant foods daily. Select the nutrient-dense and highly nutritious plant foods recommended in this book.

▫ Use healthy cooking methods. Sautéing, roasting, baking, steaming, and microwaving are all good plant-based methods. Lower heat (medium or less) and slow cooking are the best for retaining food nutrients in animal foods.

▫ Add healthy flavor to your meals. Herbs, spices, citrus, and vinegar are all great choices that add flavor. You don't need salt and sugar to make meals tasty.

▫ Try bowl meals. These meals can be highly nutritious, are cheap to make, and can provide healthy leftovers.

• **Consider the meals described in this book.** As described above, these meals will get you very close to full daily nutrition. Modify these to your own tastes but be wary of adding high levels of unhealthy ingredients. There are tons of delicious recipes using these same foods online.

• **Use the nutrition facts labels on foods.** Yes, I had to say this one last time! Please read them when selecting new foods.

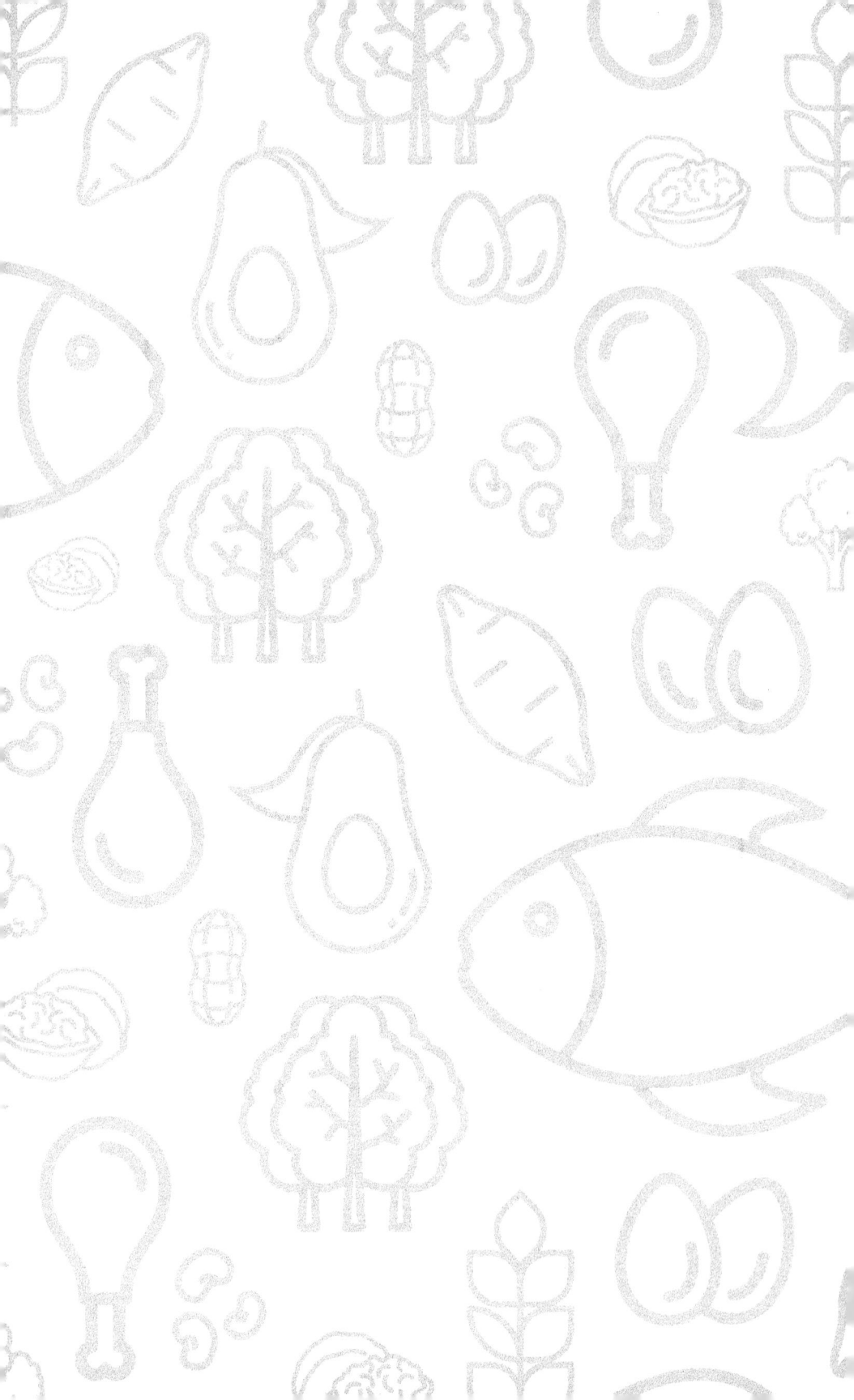

FINAL THOUGHTS

Congratulations, you have completed the book! I hope it's helped you gain a better understanding of good nutrition and how to achieve it. Good luck on your journey to a new way of eating.

Once you have made this new diet part of your routine, I believe you will be surprised how delicious the foods become. Over time, you will likely experience increased energy levels, an improved mood, and a general feeling of good health.

If you have questions or any comments on the book, please feel free to visit my website at absolutenutritionbook.com or email me directly at chris@absolutenutritionbook.com. I'd love to hear from you.

I wish you great health and delicious, nutritious eating!

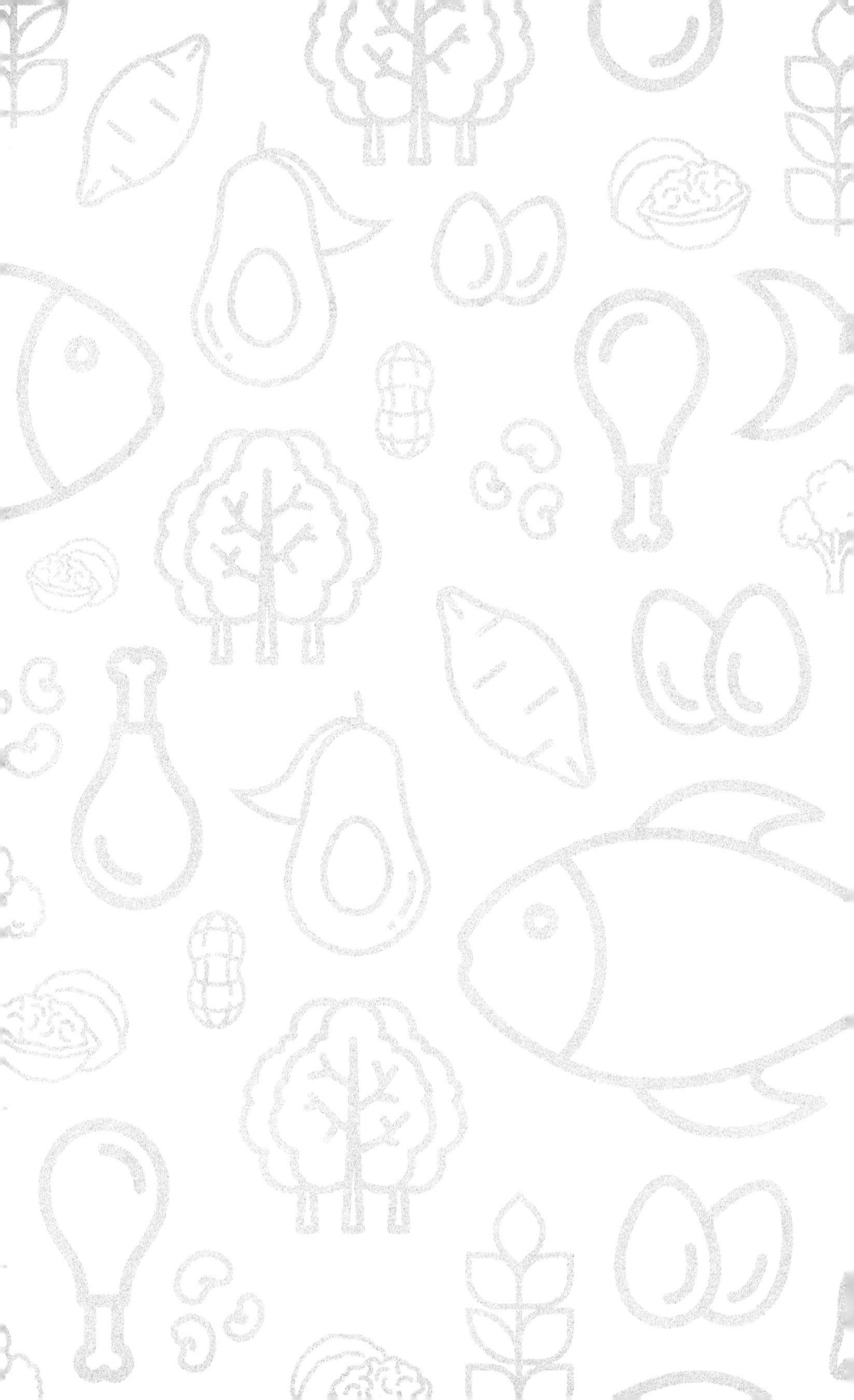

ENDNOTES

1   Miller, Jen A. "American Diets Have a Long Way to
    Go to Achieve Health Equity." *Tufts Now*, June 17, 2024. https://now.tufts.
    edu/2024/06/17/american-diets-have-long-way-go-achieve-health-equity.

2   Menichetti, Giulia, Babak Ravandi, Dariush Mozaffarian, and Albert-László
    Barabási. "Machine Learning Prediction of the Degree of Food Process-
    ing." *Nature Communications* 14 (2023): 2312. https://doi.org/10.1038/
    s41467-023-37457-1.

3   Columbia University Mailman School of Public Health. "How Long
    Do You Want to Live? Your Expectations For Old Age Matter." News.
    August 25, 2016. https://www.publichealth.columbia.edu/news/
    how-long-do-you-want-live-your-expectations-old-age-matter.

4   Lang, Frieder R., and Fiona S. Rupprecht. "Motivation for Longevity Across the
    Life Span: An Emerging Issue." *Innovation in Aging* 3, no. 2 (2019): igz014. https://
    doi.org/10.1093/geroni/igz014.

5   Thomson, Jessica, Alicia Landry, and Tameka Walls. "Can United States Adults
    Accurately Assess Their Diet Quality?" *Current Developments in Nutrition* 6, suppl. 1
    (2022): 952. https://doi.org/10.1093/cdn/nzac067.072.

6   Berg, Sara. "What Doctors Wish Patients Knew about Ultraprocessed
    Foods." *AMA*, November 8, 2024. https://www.ama-assn.org/public-health/
    prevention-wellness/what-doctors-wish-patients-knew-about-ultraprocessed-foods.

7   American Heart Association. "How Much Sugar Is Too Much?" Last reviewed
    September 23, 2024. https://www.heart.org/en/healthy-living/healthy-eating/
    eat-smart/sugar/how-much-sugar-is-too-much.

8   Centers for Disease Control and Prevention. "About Chronic Diseases."
    Last modified October 4, 2024. https://www.cdc.gov/chronic-disease/
    about/index.html.

9   Hacker, Karen. "The Burden of Chronic Disease." *Mayo Clinic Proceedings:
    Innovations, Quality & Outcomes* 8, no. 1 (2024): 112–19. https://doi.org/10.1016/j.
    mayocpiqo.2023.08.005.

10   Kim, Ju Young. "Optimal Diet Strategies for Weight Loss and Weight Loss Maintenance." *Journal of Obesity & Metabolic Syndrome* 30, no. 1 (2020): 20–31. https://doi.org/10.7570/jomes20065.

11   Cena, Hellas, and Philip C. Calder. "Defining a Healthy Diet: Evidence for the Role of Contemporary Dietary Patterns in Health and Disease." *Nutrients* 12, no. 2 (2020): 334. https://doi.org/10.3390/nu12020334.

12   Mayo Clinic. "Are High-Protein Diets Safe for Weight Loss?" April 25, 2025. https://www.mayoclinic.org/healthy-lifestyle/nutrition-and-healthy-eating/expert-answers/high-protein-diets/faq-20058207.

13   Sandoiu, Ana. "Low-Carb Diets 'Are Unsafe and Should Be Avoided.'" *Medical News Today*, August 28, 2018. https://www.medicalnewstoday.com/articles/322881#Why-low-carb-diets-should-be-avoided.

14   Alt, Kurt W., Ali Al-Ahmad, and Johan Peter Woelber. "Nutrition and Health in Human Evolution–Past to Present." *Nutrients* 14, no. 17 (2022): 3594. https://doi.org/10.3390/nu14173594.

15   Mozaffarian, Dariush, Irwin Rosenberg, and Ricardo Uauy. "History of Modern Nutrition Science—Implications for Current Research, Dietary Guidelines, and Food Policy." *BMJ* 361 (2018): k2392. https://doi.org/10.1136/bmj.k2392.

16   Thursby, Elizabeth, and Nathalie Juge. "Introduction to the Human Gut Microbiota." *Biochemical Journal* 474, no. 11 (2017): 1823–36. https://doi.org/10.1042/BCJ20160510.

17   Valdes, Ana M., Jens Walter, Eran Segal, and Tim D. Spector. "Role of the Gut Microbiota in Nutrition and Health." *BMJ* 361 (2018): k2179. https://doi.org/10.1136/bmj.k2179.

18   Wells, Diana. "19 Fun Facts About the Digestive System." *Healthline*, May 23, 2017. https://www.healthline.com/health/fun-facts-about-the-digestive-system.

19   Harvard T.H. Chan School of Public Health. "Protein." The Nutrition Source. Accessed September 30, 2025. https://nutritionsource.hsph.harvard.edu/what-should-you-eat/protein/.

20   Halton, Thomas L., and Frank B. Hu. "The Effects of High Protein Diets on Thermogenesis, Satiety and Weight Loss: A Critical Review." *Journal of the American College of Nutrition* 23, no. 5 (2004): 373–85. https://doi.org/10.1080/07315724.2004.10719381.

21   Westerterp-Plantenga, M. S., M. P. G. M. Lejeune, I. Nijs, M. van Ooijen, and E. M. R. Kovacs. "High Protein Intake Sustains Weight Maintenance after Body Weight Loss in Humans." *International Journal of Obesity* 28 (2004): 57–64. https://doi.org/10.1038/sj.ijo.0802461.

22   Cleveland Clinic. "Carbohydrates." Last reviewed March 8, 2024. https://my.clevelandclinic.org/health/articles/15416-carbohydrates.

23   MDVIP. "5 Facts About Metabolism that are Misunderstood." Accessed September 30, 2025. https://www.mdvip.com/about-mdvip/blog/five-misunderstood-facts-about-metabolism.

24   Harvard Health Publishing. "The Truth about Metabolism." July 23, 2024. https://www.health.harvard.edu/staying-healthy/the-truth-about-metabolism.

25   Tarlach, Gemma. "20 Things You Didn't Know About ... Metabolism." *Discover*, February 6, 2017. https://www.discovermagazine.com/20-things-you-didnt-know-about-metabolism-17849.

26   Mergenthaler, Philipp, Ute Lindauer, Gerald A. Dienel, and Andreas Meisel. "Sugar for the Brain: The Role of Glucose in Physiological and Pathological Brain Function." *Trends in Neurosciences* 36, no. 10 (2013): 587–97. https://doi.org/10.1016/j.tins.2013.07.001.

27   Michaud, Mark. "Study Reveals Brain's Finely Tuned System of Energy Supply." University of Rochester Medical Center News, August 7, 2016. https://www.urmc.rochester.edu/news/story/study-reveals-brains-finely-tuned-system-of-energy-supply.

28   Drake, Victoria J. "Micronutrient Inadequacies in the U.S. Population: An Overview." Linus Pauling Institute, Oregon State University. November 2017. https://lpi.oregonstate.edu/mic/micronutrient-inadequacies/overview.

29   Tardy, Anne-Laure, Etienne Pouteau, Daniel Marquez, Cansu Yilmaz, and Andrew Scholey. "Vitamins and Minerals for Energy, Fatigue and Cognition: A Narrative Review of the Biochemical and Clinical Evidence." *Nutrients* 12, no. 1 (2020): 228. https://doi.org/10.3390/nu12010228.

30   Lobo, Vijaya Chavan, A. Patil, A. Phatak, and N. Chandra. "Free Radicals, Antioxidants and Functional Foods: Impact on Human Health." *Pharmacognosy Reviews* 4, no. 8 (2010): 118–26. https://doi.org/10.4103/0973-7847.70902.

31   Eske, Jamie. "How Does Oxidative Stress Affect the Body?" *Medical News Today*, February 18, 2025. https://www.medicalnewstoday.com/articles/324863.

32   Zehiroglu, Cuma, and Sevim Beyza Ozturk Sarikaya. "The Importance of Antioxidants and Place in Today's Scientific and Technological Studies." *Journal of Food Science and Technology* 56, no. 11 (2019): 4757–74. https://doi.org/10.1007/s13197-019-03952-x.

33   Tan, Bee Ling, Mohd Esa Norhaizan, Winnie-Pui-Pui Liew, and Heshu Sulaiman Rahman. "Antioxidant and Oxidative Stress: A Mutual Interplay in Age-Related Diseases." *Frontiers in Pharmacology* 9 (2018): 1162. https://doi.org/10.3389/fphar.2018.01162.

34   Moore, Justin Xavier, Ninad Chaudhary, and Tomi Akinyemiju. "Metabolic
      Syndrome Prevalence by Race/Ethnicity and Sex in the United States, National
      Health and Nutrition Examination Survey, 1988–2012." *Preventing Chronic Disease*
      14 (2017): 160287. https://doi.org/10.5888/pcd14.160287.

35   Fryar, Cheryl D., Margaret D. Carroll, and Joseph Afful. "Prevalence of
      Overweight, Obesity, and Severe Obesity Among Adults Aged 20 and Over:
      United States, 1960–1962 Through 2017–2018." Centers for Disease Control
      and Prevention, Division of Health and Nutrition Examination Surveys. Revised
      January 29, 2021. https://www.cdc.gov/nchs/data/hestat/obesity-adult-17-18/
      obesity-adult.htm#table.

36   Soans, Rohit. "How Obesity and Diabetes Are Linked." Temple Health, May 6,
      2020. https://www.templehealth.org/about/blog/how-obesity-diabetes-are-linked
      .

37   Harvard T.H. Chan School of Public Health. "Nutrition and Immunity." The
      Nutrition Source. Accessed September 30, 2025. https://nutritionsource.hsph.
      harvard.edu/nutrition-and-immunity/.

38   Cleveland Clinic. "Immune System." Last reviewed October 20, 2023. https://
      my.clevelandclinic.org/health/body/21196-immune-system.

39   Mayo Clinic. "Chronic Inflammation: What It Is, Why It's Bad, and How You
      Can Reduce It." January 3, 2024. https://mcpress.mayoclinic.org/dairy-health/
      chronic-inflammation-what-it-is-why-its-bad-and-how-you-can-reduce-it/.

40   Munteanu, Camelia, and Betty Schwartz. "The Relationship between Nutrition
      and the Immune System." *Frontiers in Nutrition* 9 (2022): 1082500. https://doi.
      org/10.3389/fnut.2022.1082500.

41   Cherayil, Bobby J. "Iron and Immunity: Immunological Consequences of Iron
      Deficiency and Overload." *Archivum Immunologiae et Therapiae Experimentalis* 58, no. 6
      (2010): 407–15. https://doi.org/10.1007/s00005-010-0095-9.

42   Williamson, Laura. "Obesity Harms Brain Health throughout Life
      – Yet Scientists Don't Know Why." *American Heart Association News*,
      January 12, 2022. https://www.heart.org/en/news/2022/01/12/
      obesity-harms-brain-health-throughout-life-yet-scientists-dont-know-why.

43   Cleveland Clinic. "Obesity." Last reviewed September 10, 2024. https://
      my.clevelandclinic.org/health/diseases/11209-weight-control-and-obesity.

44   Beslay, Marie, Bernard Srour, Caroline Méjean, et al. "Ultra-processed Food
      Intake in Association with BMI Change and Risk of Overweight and Obesity:
      A Prospective Analysis of the French NutriNet-Santé Cohort." *PLOS Medicine* 17,
      no. 8 (2020): e1003256. https://doi.org/10.1371/journal.pmed.1003256.

45   Berg, Sara. "What Doctors Wish Patients Knew about Ultraprocessed Foods."

46   Office of Dietary Supplements, National Institutes of Health. "Nutrient Recommendations and Databases." Accessed September 30, 2025. https://ods.od.nih.gov/HealthInformation/nutrientrecommendations.aspx.

47   Murphy, Suzanne P., Allison A. Yates, Stephanie A. Atkinson, Susan I. Barr, and Johanna Dwyer. "History of Nutrition: The Long Road Leading to the Dietary Reference Intakes for the United States and Canada." *Advances in Nutrition* 7, no. 1 (2016): 157–68. https://doi.org/10.3945/an.115.010322.

48   Baum, Jamie I., Il-Young Kim, and Robert R. Wolfe. "Protein Consumption and the Elderly: What Is the Optimal Level of Intake?" *Nutrients* 8, no. 6 (2016): 359. https://doi.org/10.3390/nu8060359.

49   Godman, Heidi. "Protein Intake Associated with Less Cognitive Decline." *Harvard Health*, June 1, 2022. https://www.health.harvard.edu/mind-and-mood/protein-intake-associated-with-less-cognitive-decline.

50   Sarafrazi, Neda, Edwina A. Wambogo, and John A. Shepherd. "Osteoporosis or Low Bone Mass in Older Adults: United States, 2017–2018." *NCHS Data Brief*, no. 405, March 2021. https://www.cdc.gov/nchs/products/databriefs/db405.htm.

51   Looker, Anne C., and Chia-Yih Wang. "Prevalence of Reduced Muscle Strength in Older U.S. Adults: United States, 2011–2012." *NCHS Data Brief*, no. 179, January 2015. https://www.cdc.gov/nchs/products/databriefs/db179.htm.

52   University of Washington. "Brain Facts and Figures." Accessed September 30, 2025. https://faculty.washington.edu/chudler/facts.html.

53   Campbell, Bill, Richard B. Kreider, Tim Ziegenfuss, et al. "International Society of Sports Nutrition Position Stand: Protein and Exercise." *Journal of the International Society of Sports Nutrition* 4 (2007): 8. https://doi.org/10.1186/1550-2783-4-8.

54   University of Hawai'i at Mānoa Food Science and Human Nutrition Program. "Defining Protein." In *Human Nutrition*. University of Hawai'i at Mānoa, 2017. https://pressbooks-dev.oer.hawaii.edu/humannutrition/chapter/defining-protein/.

55   Harvard T.H. Chan School of Public Health. "Protein."

56   National Library of Medicine. "What Are Proteins and What Do They Do?" Accessed September 30, 2025. https://medlineplus.gov/genetics/understanding/howgeneswork/protein/.

57   Wempen, Kristi. "Are You Getting Enough Protein?" *Mayo Clinic Health System*, November 27, 2024. https://www.mayoclinichealthsystem.org/hometown-health/speaking-of-health/are-you-getting-too-much-protein.

58   Wolfe, Robert R., Amy M. Cifelli, Georgia Kostas, and Il-Young Kim. "Optimizing Protein Intake in Adults: Interpretation and Application of the Recommended Dietary Allowance Compared with the Acceptable Macronutrient Distribution

Range." *Advances in Nutrition* 8, no. 2 (2017): 266–75. https://doi.org/10.3945/
an.116.013821.

59   Carbone, John W., and Stefan M. Pasiakos. "Dietary Protein and Muscle Mass:
Translating Science to Application and Health Benefit." *Nutrients* 11, no. 5 (2019):
1136. https://doi.org/10.3390/nu11051136.

60   Layman, Donald K. "Dietary Guidelines Should Reflect New Understandings
about Adult Protein Needs." *Nutrition & Metabolism* 6 (2009): 12. https://doi.
org/10.1186/1743-7075-6-12.

61   Rush, Tom. "Protein Intake — How Much Protein Should You Eat Per
Day?" Healthline, April 30, 2025. https://www.healthline.com/nutrition/
how-much-protein-per-day.

62   Elango, Rajavel, Mohammad A. Humayun, Ronald O. Ball, and Paul B.
Pencharz. "Evidence that Protein Requirements Have Been Significantly Under-
estimated." *Current Opinion in Clinical Nutrition and Metabolic Care* 13, no. 1 (2010):
52–57. https://doi.org/10.1097/MCO.0b013e328332f9b7.

63   Wessels, Dan. "What Is the Average Weight for Women?" *Medical News Today*,
November 30, 2023. https://www.medicalnewstoday.com/articles/321003.

64   Gill, Stephen. "Ideal Weight Using Body Mass Index." *Medical News Today*, August
10, 2024. https://www.medicalnewstoday.com/articles/320917#ideal-weight.

65   Fryar, Cheryl D., Brian Kit, Margaret D. Carroll, and Joseph Afful. "Hyperten-
sion Prevalence, Awareness, Treatment, and Control Among Adults Age 18 and
Older: United States, August 2021–August 2023." *NCHS Data Brief*, no. 511,
October 2024. https://www.cdc.gov/nchs/products/databriefs/db511.htm.

66   Centers for Disease Control and Prevention. "Heart Disease Facts." Last
modified October 24, 2024. https://www.cdc.gov/heart-disease/data-research/
facts-stats/index.html.

67   U.S. Department of Agriculture and U.S. Department of Health and
Human Services. *Dietary Guidelines for Americans, 2020-2025*. 9th ed. December
2020. https://www.dietaryguidelines.gov/sites/default/files/2021-03/
Dietary_Guidelines_for_Americans-2020-2025.pdf.

68   American Diabetes Association. "Fats." Food & Nutrition. Accessed September
30, 2025. https://diabetes.org/food-nutrition/reading-food-labels/fats.

69   National Heart, Lung, and Blood Institute. "High Blood Triglycerides." Last modified April 19, 2023. https://www.nhlbi.nih.gov/health/
high-blood-triglycerides.

70   MacLean, P. S., J. A. Higgins, E. D. Giles, V. D. Sherk, and M. R. Jackman. "The
Role for Adipose Tissue in Weight Regain after Weight Loss." *Obesity Reviews* 16,
suppl. 1 (2015): 45–54. https://doi.org/10.1111/obr.12255.

71   Heart UK. "Saturated Fat." Accessed September 30, 2025. https://www.heartuk. org.uk/low-cholesterol-foods/saturated-fat.

72   Centers for Disease Control and Prevention. "High Cholesterol Facts." Last modified October 24, 2024. https://www.cdc.gov/cholesterol/data-research/ facts-stats/index.html.

73   Field, Catherine J., and Lindsay Robinson. "Dietary Fats." *Advances in Nutrition* 10, no. 4 (2019): 722–24. https://doi.org/10.1093/advances/nmz052.

74   Wang, Dong D., Yanping Li, Stephanie E. Chiuve, et al. "Association of Specific Dietary Fats With Total and Cause-Specific Mortality." *JAMA Internal Medicine* 176, no. 8 (2016): 1134–45. https://doi.org/10.1001/jamainternmed.2016.2417.

75   Dighriri, Ibrahim M., Abdalaziz M. Alsubaie, Fatimah M. Hakami, et al. "Effects of Omega-3 Polyunsaturated Fatty Acids on Brain Functions: A Systematic Review." *Cureus* 14, no. 10 (2022): e30091. https://doi.org/10.7759/ cureus.30091.

76   Harvard Health Publishing. "No Need to Avoid Healthy Omega-6 Fats." August 20, 2019. https://www.health.harvard.edu/newsletter_article/ no-need-to-avoid-healthy-omega-6-fats.

77   American Heart Association. "Saturated Fat." Last reviewed August 23, 2024. https://www.heart.org/en/healthy-living/healthy-eating/eat-smart/fats/ saturated-fats.

78   Williamson, Laura. "Are You Getting Enough Omega-3 Fatty Acids?" *American Heart Association News*, June 30, 2023. https://www.heart.org/en/ news/2023/06/30/are-you-getting-enough-omega-3-fatty-acids.

79   Harris, William S., Dariush Mozaffarian, Eric Rimm, et al. "Omega-6 Fatty Acids and Risk for Cardiovascular Disease: A Science Advisory From the American Heart Association Nutrition Subcommittee of the Council on Nutrition, Physical Activity, and Metabolism; Council on Cardiovascular Nursing; and Council on Epidemiology and Prevention." *Circulation* 119, no. 6 (2009): 902–7. https://doi. org/10.1161/CIRCULATIONAHA.108.191627.

80   American Heart Association News. "Consuming about 3 Grams of Omega-3 Fatty Acids a Day May Lower Blood Pressure." *American Heart Association News*, June 1, 2022. https://www.heart.org/en/news/2022/06/01/ consuming-about-3-grams-of-omega-3-fatty-acids-a-day-may- lower-blood-pressure.

81   Office of Dietary Supplements, National Institutes of Health. "Omega-3 Fatty Acids: Fact Sheet for Consumers." Updated July 18, 2022. https://ods.od.nih. gov/factsheets/Omega3FattyAcids-Consumer/.

82   Harvard Health Publishing. "Know the Facts about Fats." April 19, 2021. https://www.health.harvard.edu/staying-healthy/know-the-facts-about-fats.

83   Harvard Health Publishing. "Understanding Triglycerides." July 24, 2023. https://www.health.harvard.edu/heart-health/understanding-triglycerides.

84   Cox, Rafael A., and Mario R. García-Palmieri. "Cholesterol, Triglycerides, and Associated Lipoproteins." In *Clinical Methods: The History, Physical, and Laboratory Examinations*, 3rd ed., edited by H. K. Walker, W. D. Hall, and J. W. Hurst. Butterworths, 1990. https://www.ncbi.nlm.nih.gov/books/NBK351/.

85   McDonell, Kayla. "Why Dietary Cholesterol Does Not Matter (For Most People)." Healthline, September 15, 2023. https://www.healthline.com/nutrition/dietary-cholesterol-does-not-matter.

86   Field, Catherine J., and Lindsay Robinson. "Dietary Fats."

87   Berry, Jennifer. "Polyunsaturated Fat: Everything You Need to Know." *Medical News Today*, February 11, 2020. https://www.medicalnewstoday.com/articles/polyunsaturated-fat#benefits.

88   Hjalmarsdottir, Freydis. "The 3 Most Important Types of Omega-3 Fatty Acids." *Healthline*, May 27, 2019. https://www.healthline.com/nutrition/3-types-of-omega-3.

89   DiNicolantonio, James J., and James H. O'Keefe. "The Importance of Marine Omega-3s for Brain Development and the Prevention and Treatment of Behavior, Mood, and Other Brain Disorders." *Nutrients* 12, no. 8 (2020): 2333. https://doi.org/10.3390/nu12082333.

90   Djuricic, Ivana, and Philip C. Calder. "Beneficial Outcomes of Omega-6 and Omega-3 Polyunsaturated Fatty Acids on Human Health: An Update for 2021." *Nutrients* 13, no. 7 (2021): 2421. https://doi.org/10.3390/nu13072421.

91   Nature Publishing Group. "Can One Gram of Omega-3 Really Slow Aging? Here's What Science Says." *SciTechDaily*, April 30, 2025. https://scitechdaily.com/can-one-gram-of-omega-3-really-slow-aging-heres-what-science-says/.

92   "Healthy Foods High in Omega-6." *WebMD*, October 17, 2024. https://www.webmd.com/diet/foods-high-in-omega-6.

93   Schwingshackl, Lukas, and Georg Hoffmann. "Monounsaturated Fatty Acids, Olive Oil and Health Status: A Systematic Review and Meta-analysis of Cohort Studies." *Lipids in Health and Disease* 13 (2014): 154. https://doi.org/10.1186/1476-511X-13-154.

94   American Heart Association. "Monounsaturated Fats." Last reviewed October 25, 2023. https://www.heart.org/en/healthy-living/healthy-eating/eat-smart/fats/monounsaturated-fats.

95   Mayo Clinic. "Trans Fat Is Double Trouble for Heart Health." February 1, 2025. https://www.mayoclinic.org/diseases-conditions/high-blood-cholesterol/in-depth/trans-fat/art-20046114.

96   Harvard T.H. Chan School of Public Health. " Types of Fat." The Nutrition Source. Accessed September 30, 2025. https://nutritionsource.hsph.harvard.edu/what-should-you-eat/fats-and-cholesterol/types-of-fat/.

97   U.S. Department of Agriculture and U.S. Department of Health and Human Services. *Dietary Guidelines for Americans, 2020-2025*. 9th ed.

98   Centers for Disease Control and Prevention. "Type 2 Diabetes." Last modified May 15, 2024. https://www.cdc.gov/diabetes/about/about-type-2-diabetes.html.

99   Centers for Disease Control and Prevention. "1 in 3 Americans Have Prediabetes Social Media Graphic." Last modified May 15, 2024. https://www.cdc.gov/diabetes/communication-resources/1-in-3-americans.html.

100   Pinhas-Hamiel, Orit, and Philip Zeitler. "Type 2 Diabetes in Children and Adolescents- A Focus on Diagnosis and Treatment." In *Endotext*, edited by K. R. Feingold, S. F. Ahmed, B. Anawalt, et al. MDText.com, Inc., 2000-. Last updated November 7, 2023. https://www.ncbi.nlm.nih.gov/books/NBK597439/.

101   Caputo, Joseph. "Study Links Poor Diet to 14 Million Cases of Type 2 Diabetes Globally." *Tufts Now*, April 17, 2023. https://now.tufts.edu/2023/04/17/study-links-poor-diet-14-million-cases-type-2-diabetes-globally.

102   U.S. Department of Agriculture, Agricultural Research Service. "FoodData Central." Accessed September 30, 2025. https://fdc.nal.usda.gov/.

103   Cleveland Clinic. "Carbohydrates." Last reviewed March 8, 2024. https://my.clevelandclinic.org/health/articles/15416-carbohydrates.

104   McKeown, Nicola M., George C. Fahey Jr., Joanne Slavin, and Jan-Willem van der Kamp. "Fibre Intake for Optimal Health: How Can Healthcare Professionals Support People to Reach Dietary Recommendations?" *BMJ* 378 (2022): e054370. https://doi.org/10.1136/bmj-2020-054370.

105   Quagliani, Diane, and Patricia Felt-Gunderson. "Closing America's Fiber Intake Gap: Communication Strategies From a Food and Fiber Summit." *American Journal of Lifestyle Medicine* 11, no. 1 (2016): 80–85. https://doi.org/10.1177/1559827615588079.

106   Harvard Health Publishing. "The Sweet Danger of Sugar." January 6, 2022. https://www.health.harvard.edu/heart-health/the-sweet-danger-of-sugar.

107   Gunnars, Kris. "Carbohydrates: Whole vs. Refined — Here's the Difference." *Healthline*, February 2, 2023. https://www.healthline.com/nutrition/good-carbs-bad-carbs.

108   Kubala, Jillian. "11 Reasons Why Too Much Sugar Is Bad for You." *Healthline*, November 27, 2024. https://www.healthline.com/nutrition/too-much-sugar.

109   Soler Rivera, Luis. "Effects of Sugar on the Brain: Cravings and Inflammation." UVA Health, January 15, 2020. https://blog.uvahealth.com/2020/01/15/effects-sugar-brain/.

110   Huang, Yin, Zeyu Chen, Bo Chen, et al. "Dietary Sugar Consumption and Health: Umbrella Review." *BMJ* 381 (2023): e071609. https://doi.org/10.1136/bmj-2022-071609.

111   University of Rochester Medical Center. "The Truth About Triglycerides." Accessed September 30, 2025. https://www.urmc.rochester.edu/encyclopedia/content?contenttypeid=56&contentid=2967.

112   American Heart Association. "Added Sugars." Last reviewed August 2, 2024. https://www.heart.org/en/healthy-living/healthy-eating/eat-smart/sugar/added-sugars.

113   Gunnars, Kris. "How Much Sugar Should You Eat Per Day?" *Healthline*, November 6, 2024. https://www.healthline.com/nutrition/how-much-sugar-per-day#faq.

114   Brazier, Yvette. "What Are Vitamins, and How Do They Work?" *Medical News Today*, October 5, 2023. https://www.medicalnewstoday.com/articles/195878.

115   Harvard Health Publishing. "Precious Metals and Other Important Minerals for Health." February 15, 2021. https://www.health.harvard.edu/staying-healthy/precious-metals-and-other-important-minerals-for-health.

116   Drake, Victoria J. "Micronutrient Inadequacies in the U.S. Population: An Overview."

117   Reider, Carroll A., Ray-Yuan Chung, Prasad P. Devarshi, Ryan W. Grant, and Susan Hazels Mitmesser. "Inadequacy of Immune Health Nutrients: Intakes in U.S. Adults, the 2005–2016 NHANES." *Nutrients* 12, no. 6 (2020): 1735. https://doi.org/10.3390/nu12061735.

118   Ho, Emily. "Zinc Deficiencies a Global Concern." Oregon State University News, September 17, 2009. https://news.oregonstate.edu/news/zinc-deficiencies-global-concern.

119   Baik, H. W., and R. M. Russell. "Vitamin B12 Deficiency in the Elderly." *Annual Review of Nutrition* 19 (1999): 357–77. https://doi.org/10.1146/annurev.nutr.19.1.357.

120   Hoy, M. Katherine, Joseph D. Goldman, and Alanna Moshfegh. "Potassium Intake of the U.S. Population: What We Eat in America, NHANES 2017-2018." In *FSRG Dietary Data Briefs*, Dietary Data Brief No. 47. U.S. Department of Agriculture, September 2022. https://www.ncbi.nlm.nih.gov/books/NBK587683/.

121   Harth, Richard. "Study Explores Effects of Dietary Choline Deficiency on Neurologic, Systemwide Health." Arizona State University News, January 17, 2023. https://news.asu.edu/20230117-study-explores-effects-dietary-choline-deficiency-neurologic-systemwide-health.

122   Weyand, Angela C., Alexander Chaitoff, Gary L. Freed, Michelle Sholzberg, Sung Won Choi, and Patrick T. McGann. "Prevalence of Iron Deficiency and Iron-Deficiency Anemia in U.S. Females Aged 12-21 Years, 2003-2020." *JAMA* 329, no. 24 (2023): 2191–93. https://doi.org/10.1001/jama.2023.8020.

123   U.S. Food and Drug Administration. "Sodium in Your Diet." Content current as of March 5, 2024. https://www.fda.gov/food/nutrition-education-resources-materials/sodium-your-diet.

124   Office of Dietary Supplements, National Institutes of Health. "For Health Professionals." Accessed September 30, 2025. https://ods.od.nih.gov/HealthInformation/healthprofessional.aspx.

125   Institute of Medicine (U.S.) Panel on Dietary Antioxidants and Related Compounds. *Dietary Reference Intakes for Vitamin C, Vitamin E, Selenium, and Carotenoids*. National Academies Press, 2000. https://www.ncbi.nlm.nih.gov/books/NBK225480/.

126   Carr, Anitra C., and Silvia Maggini. "Vitamin C and Immune Function." *Nutrients* 9, no. 11 (2017): 1211. https://doi.org/10.3390/nu9111211.

127   Cleveland Clinic. "Should You Take Iron With Vitamin C?" December 8, 2023. https://health.clevelandclinic.org/iron-and-vitamin-c.

128   Hanna, Mary, Ecler Jaqua, Van Nguyen, and Jeremy Clay. "B Vitamins: Functions and Uses in Medicine." *Permanente Journal* 26, no. 2 (2022): 89–97. https://doi.org/10.7812/TPP/21.204.

129   Olaso-Gonzalez, Gloria, Marco Inzitari, Giuseppe Bellelli, Alessandro Morandi, Núria Barcons, and José Viña. "Impact of Supplementation with Vitamins B6, B12, and/or Folic Acid on the Reduction of Homocysteine Levels in Patients with Mild Cognitive Impairment: A Systematic Review." *IUBMB Life* 74, no. 1 (2022): 74–84. https://doi.org/10.1002/iub.2507.

130   Martinaityte, Ieva, Elena Kamycheva, Allan Didriksen, Jette Jakobsen, and Rolf Jorde. "Vitamin D Stored in Fat Tissue During a 5-Year Intervention Affects Serum 25-Hydroxyvitamin D Levels the Following Year." *Journal of Clinical Endocrinology & Metabolism* 102, no. 10 (2017): 3731–38. https://doi.org/10.1210/jc.2017-01187.

131   Raman, Ryan. "How to Safely Get Vitamin D From Sunlight." *Healthline*, November 26, 2024. https://www.healthline.com/nutrition/vitamin-d-from-sun.

132   American Osteopathic Association. "Researchers Find Low Magnesium Levels Make Vitamin D Ineffective." Accessed September 30, 2025. https://findado.osteopathic.org/researchers-find-low-magnesium-levels-make-vitamin-d-ineffective.

133   Meydani, Simin Nikbin, Lynette S. Leka, Basil C. Fine, et al. "Vitamin E and Respiratory Tract Infections in Elderly Nursing Home Residents: A Randomized Controlled Trial." *JAMA* 292, no. 7 (2004): 828–36. https://doi.org/10.1001/jama.292.7.828.

134   Michels, Alexander J. "Vitamin E and Skin Health." Linus Pauling Institute, Oregon State University. February 2012. https://lpi.oregonstate.edu/mic/health-disease/skin-health/vitamin-E.

135   Klein, Eric A., Ian M. Thompson, Catherine M. Tangen, et al. "Vitamin E and the Risk of Prostate Cancer: The Selenium and Vitamin E Cancer Prevention Trial (**SELECT**)." *JAMA* 306, no. 14 (2011): 1549–56. https://doi.org/10.1001/jama.2011.1437.

136   Harvard T.H. Chan School of Public Health. "Vitamin A." The Nutrition Source. Accessed September 30, 2025. https://nutritionsource.hsph.harvard.edu/vitamin-a/.

137   Huang, Zhiyi, Yu Liu, Guangying Qi, David Brand, and Song Guo Zheng. "Role of Vitamin A in the Immune System." *Journal of Clinical Medicine* 7, no. 9 (2018): 258. https://doi.org/10.3390/jcm7090258.

138   Wu, Juan, Eunyoung Cho, Walter C. Willett, Srinivas M. Sastry, and Debra A. Schaumberg. "Intakes of Lutein, Zeaxanthin, and Other Carotenoids and Age-Related Macular Degeneration During 2 Decades of Prospective Follow-up." *JAMA Ophthalmology* 133, no. 12 (2015): 1415–24. https://doi.org/10.1001/jamaophthalmol.2015.3590.

139   Drake, Victoria J. "Vitamin K." Linus Pauling Institute, Oregon State University. Updated May 2022. https://lpi.oregonstate.edu/mic/vitamins/vitamin-K.

140   Derbyshire, Emma. "Could We Be Overlooking a Potential Choline Crisis in the United Kingdom?" *BMJ Nutrition, Prevention & Health* 2, no. 2 (2019): 86–89. https://doi.org/10.1136/bmjnph-2019-000037.

141   University of Rochester Medical Center. "Zinc." Health Encyclopedia. Accessed September 30, 2025. https://www.urmc.rochester.edu/encyclopedia/content?contenttypeid=19&contentid=zinc.

142   Prasad, Ananda S. "Zinc: An Antioxidant and Anti-inflammatory Agent: Role of Zinc in Degenerative Disorders of Aging." *Journal of Trace Elements in Medicine and Biology* 28, no. 4 (2014): 364–71. https://doi.org/10.1016/j.jmb.2014.04.006.

143 "Foods High in Zinc." WebMD, September 24, 2024. https://www.webmd.com/diet/foods-high-in-zinc.

144 National Library of Medicine. "Fluid and Electrolyte Balance." Accessed September 30, 2025. https://medlineplus.gov/fluidandelectrolytebalance.html.

145 National Institute of Diabetes and Digestive and Kidney Diseases. "Definition & Facts for Lactose Intolerance." Last reviewed February 2018. https://www.niddk.nih.gov/health-information/digestive-diseases/lactose-intolerance/definition-facts#common.

146 Reddy, Pramod, and Linda R. Edwards. "Magnesium Supplementation in Vitamin D Deficiency." *American Journal of Therapeutics* 26, no. 1 (2019): e124–32. https://doi.org/10.1097/MJT.0000000000000538.

147 Cook, Nancy R., Feng J. He, Graham A. MacGregor, and Niels Graudal. "Sodium and Health—Concordance and Controversy." *BMJ* 369 (2020): m2440. https://doi.org/10.1136/bmj.m2440.

148 Delage, Barbara. "Sodium (Chloride)." Linus Pauling Institute, Oregon State University. Updated May 2016. https://lpi.oregonstate.edu/mic/minerals/sodium.

149 American Heart Association. "How Potassium Can Help Prevent or Treat High Blood Pressure." Last reviewed August 14, 2025. https://www.heart.org/en/health-topics/high-blood-pressure/changes-you-can-make-to-manage-high-blood-pressure/how-potassium-can-help-control-high-blood-pressure.

150 Harvard T.H. Chan School of Public Health. "Iron." The Nutrition Source. Accessed September 30, 2025. https://nutritionsource.hsph.harvard.edu/iron/.

151 Tawfik, Yahya M. K., Hayley Billingsley, Ankeet S. Bhatt, et al. "Absolute and Functional Iron Deficiency in the U.S., 2017-2020." *JAMA Network Open* 7, no. 9 (2024): e2433126. https://doi.org/10.1001/jamanetworkopen.2024.33126.

152 Metcalf, Eric. "Phytonutrients." *WebMD*, October 17, 2024. https://www.webmd.com/diet/phytonutrients-faq.

153 Fahey, Jed W., and Thomas W. Kensler. "Phytochemicals: Do They Belong on Our Plate for Sustaining Healthspan?" *Food Front* 2, no. 3 (2021): 235–39. https://doi.org/10.1002/fft2.81.

154 Ullah, Asad, Sidra Munir, Syed Lal Badshah, Noreen Khan, Lubna Ghani, Benjamin Gabriel Poulson, Abdul-Hamid Emwas, and Mariusz Jaremko. "Important Flavonoids and Their Role as a Therapeutic Agent." *Molecules* 25, no. 22 (2020): 5243. https://doi.org/10.3390/molecules25225243.

155 Haytowitz, David B., Xianli Wu, and Seema Bhagwat. *USDA Database for the Flavonoid Content of Selected Foods, Release 3.3.* U.S. Department of Agriculture,

Agricultural Research Service, Nutrient Data Laboratory, March 2018. https:// www.ars.usda.gov/ARSUserFiles/80400535/Data/Flav/Flav3.3.pdf.

156   Crupi, Pasquale, Maria Felicia Faienza, Muhammad Yasir Naeem, Filomena Corbo, Maria Lisa Clodoveo, and Marilena Muraglia. "Overview of the Potential Beneficial Effects of Carotenoids on Consumer Health and Well-Being." *Antioxidants* 12, no. 5 (2023): 1069. https://doi.org/10.3390/antiox12051069.

157   U.S. Department of Agriculture, Agricultural Research Service. *USDA National Nutrient Database for Standard Reference Release 28: Nutrients: Carotene, Beta (µg)*. October 28, 2015. https://ods.od.nih.gov/pubs/usdandb/ VitA-betaCarotene-Content.pdf.

158   U.S. Department of Agriculture, Agricultural Research Service. *USDA National Nutrient Database for Standard Reference Legacy (2018): Nutrients: Lutein + Zeaxanthin (µg)*. 2018. https://www.nal.usda.gov/sites/default/files/page-files/Lutein_ zeaxanthin.pdf.

159   U.S. Department of Agriculture, Agricultural Research Service. *USDA National Nutrient Database for Standard Reference Legacy (2018): Nutrients: Lycopene (µg)*. 2018. https://www.nal.usda.gov/sites/default/files/page-files/Lycopene.pdf.

160   Miękus, Natalia, Krystian Marszałek, Magdalena Podlacha, Aamir Iqbal, Czesław Puchalski, and Artur H. Świergiel. "Health Benefits of Plant-Derived Sulfur Compounds, Glucosinolates, and Organosulfur Compounds." *Molecules* 25, no. 17 (2020): 3804. https://doi.org/10.3390/molecules25173804.

161   Gambari, Laura, Brunella Grigolo, and Francesco Grassi. "Dietary Organosulfur Compounds: Emerging Players in the Regulation of Bone Homeostasis by Plant-Derived Molecules." *Frontiers in Endocrinology* 13 (2022): 937956. https://doi. org/10.3389/fendo.2022.937956.

162   Kumar, Naresh, and Nidhi Goel. "Phenolic Acids: Natural Versatile Molecules with Promising Therapeutic Applications." *Biotechnology Reports* 24 (2019): e00370. https://doi.org/10.1016/j.btre.2019.e00370.

163   Ajmera, Rachael. "Ellagic Acid: What It Is, How It Works, and Food Sources." *Healthline*, August 16, 2021. https://www.healthline.com/nutrition/ellagic-acid.

164   Godos, Justyna, Filippo Caraci, Agnieszka Micek, Sabrina Castellano, Emanuele D'Amico, Nadia Paladino, Raffaele Ferri, Fabio Galvano, and Giuseppe Grosso. "Dietary Phenolic Acids and Their Major Food Sources Are Associated with Cognitive Status in Older Italian Adults." *Antioxidants* 10, no. 5 (2021): 700. https://doi.org/10.3390/antiox10050700.

165   Neveu, V., J. Pérez-Jiménez, F. Vos, V. Crespy, L. du Chaffaut, L. Mennen, C. Knox, R. Eisner, J. Cruz, D. Wishart, and A. Scalbert. "Vanillic Acid." Phenol-Explorer, version 3.6. Accessed September 30, 2025. http:// phenol-explorer.eu/contents/polyphenol/414.

166   Neveu, V., J. Pérez-Jiménez, F. Vos, V. Crespy, L. du Chaffaut, L. Mennen, C. Knox, R. Eisner, J. Cruz, D. Wishart, and A. Scalbert. "Syringic Acid." Phenol-Explorer, version 3.6. Accessed September 30, 2025. http://phenol-explorer.eu/contents/polyphenol/420.

167   Anlar, Hatice Gül. "Cinnamic Acid as a Dietary Antioxidant in Diabetes Treatment." In *Diabetes: Oxidative Stress and Dietary Antioxidants*, 2nd ed., edited by Victor R. Preedy. Academic Press, 2020. https://doi.org/10.1016/C2017-0-03571-1.

168   Gómez-Zorita, Saioa, Maitane González-Arceo, Alfredo Fernández-Quintela, Itziar Eseberri, Jenifer Trepiana, and María Puy Portillo. "Scientific Evidence Supporting the Beneficial Effects of Isoflavones on Human Health." *Nutrients* 12, no. 12 (2020): 3853. https://doi.org/10.3390/nu12123853.

169   Bhagwat, Seema, David B. Haytowitz, and Joanne M. Holden. *USDA Database for the Isoflavone Content of Selected Foods, Release 2.0*. U.S. Department of Agriculture, Agricultural Research Service, Nutrient Data Laboratory, September 2008. http://www.ars.usda.gov/nutrientdata/isoflav.

170   Rodríguez-García, Carmen, Cristina Sánchez-Quesada, Estefanía Toledo, Miguel Delgado-Rodríguez, and José J. Gaforio. "Naturally Lignan-Rich Foods: A Dietary Tool for Health Promotion?" *Molecules* 24, no. 5 (2019): 917. https://doi.org/10.3390/molecules24050917.

171   Meng, Xiao, Jing Zhou, Cai-Ning Zhao, Ren-You Gan, and Hua-Bin Li. "Health Benefits and Molecular Mechanisms of Resveratrol: A Narrative Review." *Foods* 9, no. 3 (2020): 340. https://doi.org/10.3390/foods9030340.

172   Xu, Yichi, Mengxue Fang, Xue Li, Du Wang, Li Yu, Fei Ma, Jun Jiang, Liangxiao Zhang, and Peiwu Li. "Contributions of Common Foods to Resveratrol Intake in the Chinese Diet." *Foods* 13, no. 8 (2024): 1267. https://doi.org/10.3390/foods13081267.

173   U.S. Department of Agriculture, Agricultural Research Service. "FoodData Central Food Search." Accessed September 30, 2025. https://fdc.nal.usda.gov/food-search?type=SR%20Legacy.

174   Wessels, Dan. "What Is the Average Weight for Women?"

175   Gill, Stephen. "Is There an Average Weight for Men?" *Medical News Today*, August 10, 2024. https://www.medicalnewstoday.com/articles/320917.

176   Spritzler, Franziska. "How Cooking Affects the Nutrient Content of Foods." *Healthline*, November 7, 2019. https://www.healthline.com/nutrition/cooking-nutrient-content.

177   Giosuè, Annalisa, Ilaria Calabrese, Marilena Vitale, Gabriele Riccardi, and Olga Vaccaro. "Consumption of Dairy Foods and Cardiovascular

Disease: A Systematic Review." *Nutrients* 14, no. 4 (2022): 831. https://doi.org/10.3390/nu14040831.

178   European Society of Cardiology. "New Research Challenges Advice To Limit High-Fat Dairy Foods." *SciTechDaily*, August 23, 2023. https://scitechdaily.com/new-research-challenges-advice-to-limit-high-fat-dairy-foods/.

179   Harvard Health Publishing. "What's the Beef with Red Meat?" February 1, 2020. https://www.health.harvard.edu/staying-healthy/whats-the-beef-with-red-meat.

180   National Institutes of Health. "Eating Red Meat Daily Triples Heart Disease-Related Chemical." NIH Research Matters. January 8, 2019. https://www.nih.gov/news-events/nih-research-matters/eating-red-meat-daily-triples-heart-disease-related-chemical.

181   Cleveland Clinic. "Is Red Meat Bad for You?" February 14, 2024. https://health.clevelandclinic.org/is-red-meat-bad-for-you/.

182   U.S. Food and Drug Administration. "Advice about Eating Fish: For Those Who Might Become or Are Pregnant or Breastfeeding and Children Ages 1 - 11 Years." Content current as of March 5, 2024. https://www.fda.gov/food/consumers/advice-about-eating-fish.

183   Pearson, Keith. "Is Tilapia Good for You?" *Healthline*, October 1, 2025. https://www.healthline.com/nutrition/tilapia-fish.

184   U.S. Department of Agriculture, Agricultural Research Service. "Fast Foods, Fish Sandwich, with Tartar Sauce and Cheese." FoodData Central. Published April 1, 2019. https://fdc.nal.usda.gov/food-details/170297/nutrients.

185   Soltani, Sepideh, and Mohammadreza Vafa. "The Dairy Fat Paradox: Whole Dairy Products May Be Healthier Than We Thought." *Medical Journal of the Islamic Republic of Iran* 31 (2017): 110. https://doi.org/10.14196/mjiri.31.110.

186   Slotkin, Ellen. "Red Meat With Lower Cholesterol Impact: Incorporating Lean Cuts into a Low-Cholesterol Diet." *Verywell Health*, May 15, 2024. https://www.verywellhealth.com/low-cholesterol-food-swaps-meat-and-cholesterol-697807.

187   Nutrition Value. "BURGER KING, Cheeseburger." Accessed September 30, 2025. https://www.nutritionvalue.org/BURGER_KING%2C_Cheeseburger_nutritional_value.html.

188   Nutrition Value. "McDONALD'S, French Fries." Accessed September 30, 2025. https://www.nutritionvalue.org/McDONALD%27S%2C_french_fries_nutritional_value.html?size=1.0+medium+serving+%3D+117.0+g.

189   Eat This Much. "Cola." Accessed September 30, 2025. https://www.eatthismuch.com/calories/cola-3100?a=0.7494908350305498%3A2.

190   Watson, Stephanie. "Health Benefits of Vegetables." *WebMD*, August 27, 2024. https://www.webmd.com/diet/health-benefits-vegetables.

191   UH Hospitals. "Is Pasta Healthier When It's Eaten Cold?" December 15, 2023. https://www.uhhospitals.org/blog/articles/2023/12/is-pasta-healthier-when-its-eaten-cold.

192   Pagán, Camille Noe, and Timothy Gower. "What Are the Best Fruits for Diabetes?" *WebMD*, July 31, 2024. https://www.webmd.com/diabetes/fruit-diabetes.

193   Richa, Rishi, Deepika Kohli, Dinesh Vishwakarma, Ananya Mishra, Bhumika Kabdal, Anjineyulu Kothakota, Shruti Richa, Ranjna Sirohi, Rohitashw Kumar, and Bindu Naik. "Citrus Fruit: Classification, Value Addition, Nutritional and Medicinal Values, and Relation with Pandemic and Hidden Hunger." *Journal of Agriculture and Food Research* 14 (2023): 100718. https://doi.org/10.1016/j.jafr.2023.100718.

194   Brown, Jessica. "Frozen, Fresh or Canned Food: What's More Nutritious?" *BBC Future*, April 28, 2020. https://www.bbc.com/future/article/20200427-frozen-fresh-or-canned-food-whats-more-nutritious.

195   Brown, Mary Jane. "Fresh vs Frozen Fruit and Vegetables — Which Are Healthier?" *Healthline*, June 15, 2017. https://www.healthline.com/nutrition/fresh-vs-frozen-fruit-and-vegetables.

196   McCallum, Katie. "Are Canned & Frozen Veggies As Healthy As Fresh Ones?" Houston Methodist, March 3, 2021. https://www.houstonmethodist.org/blog/articles/2021/mar/are-canned-and-frozen-veggies-as-healthy-as-fresh-ones/.

197   American Heart Association. "Fresh, Frozen or Canned Fruit and Vegetables: All Can Be Healthy Choices." Last reviewed October 24, 2023. https://www.heart.org/en/healthy-living/healthy-eating/add-color/fresh-frozen-or-canned-fruits-and-vegetables-all-can-be-healthy-choices.

198   Wildly Organic. "How Long Do Nuts Last? Tips for Storing Nuts and Seeds." August 30, 2021. https://wildlyorganic.com/blogs/recipes/how-long-do-nuts-last-tips-for-storing-nuts-and-seeds.

199   Utah State University Extension. "Storing Dry Beans." Accessed September 30, 2025. https://extension.usu.edu/preserve-the-harvest/dev/storing-dry-beans-1.

200   Harvard T.H. Chan School of Public Health. "Legumes and Pulses." The Nutrition Source. Accessed September 30, 2025. https://nutritionsource.hsph.harvard.edu/legumes-pulses/.

201   Streit, Lizzie, and Ruairi Robertson. "9 Healthy Beans and Legumes You Should Try." *Healthline*, June 30, 2023. https://www.healthline.com/nutrition/healthiest-beans-legumes.

202   Burgess, Lana. "What Are the Nutritional Benefits of Peanuts?" *Medical News Today*, April 18, 2019. https://www.medicalnewstoday.com/articles/325003#nutrition.

203   Arya, Shalini S., Akshata R. Salve, and S. Chauhan. "Peanuts as Functional Food: A Review." *Journal of Food Science and Technology* 53, no. 1 (2015): 31–41. https://doi.org/10.1007/s13197-015-2007-9.

204   Johnson, Jon. "What Are the Most Healthful Nuts You Can Eat?" *Medical News Today*, September 11, 2018. https://www.medicalnewstoday.com/articles/323042.

205   Woźniak, Magdalena, Agnieszka Waśkiewicz, and Izabela Ratajczak. "The Content of Phenolic Compounds and Mineral Elements in Edible Nuts." *Molecules* 27, no. 14 (2022): 4326. https://doi.org/10.3390/molecules27144326.

206   National Geographic Society. "Grain." National Geographic Education. Last updated December 9, 2024. https://education.nationalgeographic.org/resource/grain/.

207   Mayo Clinic. "Whole Grains: Hearty Options for a Healthy Diet." August 19, 2025. https://www.mayoclinic.org/healthy-lifestyle/nutrition-and-healthy-eating/in-depth/whole-grains/art-20047826.

208   Cleveland Clinic. "The 6 Best Seeds to Eat." January 13, 2021. https://health.clevelandclinic.org/the-6-best-seeds-to-eat.

209   McCulloch, Marsha. "Cacao vs Cocoa: What's the Difference?" *Healthline*, July 12, 2023. https://www.healthline.com/nutrition/cacao-vs-cocoa#nutrition.

210   Mayo Clinic. "Organic Foods: Are They Safer? More Nutritious?" February 28, 2025. https://www.mayoclinic.org/healthy-lifestyle/nutrition-and-healthy-eating/in-depth/organic-food/art-20043880.

211   Harvard Health Publishing. "Should You Go Organic?" September 9, 2015. https://www.health.harvard.edu/staying-healthy/should-you-go-organic.

212   Cleveland Clinic. "Organic Foods: Are They Better for You?" May 8, 2024. https://health.clevelandclinic.org/organic-food.

213   UPMC HealthBeat. "Health Benefits of Salmon." Reviewed by Allison P. Lutz. March 11, 2024. https://share.upmc.com/2023/04/health-benefits-of-salmon/.

214   Kendall Reagan Nutrition Center. "Wild Caught vs. Farm Raised Seafood." Colorado State University, April 17, 2018. https://chhs.source.colostate.edu/wild-caught-vs-farm-raised-seafood/.

215   DiGiacinto, Jessica, and Joe Leech. "Wild vs. Farmed Salmon: Which Type of Salmon Is Healthier?" *Healthline*, September 28, 2023. https://www.healthline.com/nutrition/wild-vs-farmed-salmon.

216   "Health Benefits of Chicken." *WebMD*, September 28, 2024. https://www.
      webmd.com/diet/health-benefits-chicken.

217   Ajmera, Rachael. "Is Chicken Healthy? Nutrition, Benefits, and Tips."
      Healthline, October 20, 2020. https://www.healthline.com/nutrition/
      is-chicken-good-for-you.

218   Rubenfire, Melvyn. "Dietary Cholesterol and Cardiovascular Risk: AHA
      Advisory." American College of Cardiology, January 10, 2020. https://www.
      acc.org/latest-in-cardiology/ten-points-to-remember/2019/12/30/15/23/
      dietary-cholesterol-and-cardiovascular-risk.

219   Gunnars, Kris. "9 Benefits of Eggs." *Healthline*, December 20, 2024. https://www.
      healthline.com/nutrition/proven-health-benefits-of-eggs.

220   National Cancer Institute. "Cruciferous Vegetables and Cancer Preven-
      tion." Reviewed June 7, 2012. https://www.cancer.gov/about-cancer/
      causes-prevention/risk/diet/cruciferous-vegetables-fact-sheet.

221   Ware, Megan. "11 Health Benefits of Avocado." *Medical News Today*, July 8, 2025.
      https://www.medicalnewstoday.com/articles/270406.

222   California Fresh Fruit Association. "Mexico Continues to Lead World Avocado
      Production." April 16, 2024. https://calfruitandveg.com/2024/04/16/
      mexico-continues-to-lead-world-avocado-production.

223   Booth, Stephanie. "Health Benefits of Sweet Potatoes." *WebMD*, July 26, 2025.
      https://www.webmd.com/food-recipes/benefits-sweet-potatoes.

224   Harvard T.H. Chan School of Public Health. "Legumes and Pulses."

225   Burgess, Lana. "What Are the Nutritional Benefits of Peanuts?"

226   Arya, Shalini S., Akshata R. Salve, and S. Chauhan. "Peanuts as Functional
      Food: A Review."

227   Ros, Emilio. "Health Benefits of Nut Consumption." *Nutrients* 2, no. 7 (2010):
      652–82. https://doi.org/10.3390/nu2070652.

228   Cleveland Clinic. "The Whole Truth About Whole Grains." March 8, 2023.
      https://health.clevelandclinic.org/the-whole-truth-about-whole-grains.

229   Vahapoglu, Beyza, Ezgi Erskine, Busra Gultekin Subasi, and Esra Capanoglu.
      "Recent Studies on Berry Bioactives and Their Health-Promoting Roles."
      Molecules 27, no. 1 (2021): 108. https://doi.org/10.3390/molecules27010108.

230   Robertson, Ruairi. "6 Super Healthy Seeds You Should Eat." *Healthline*, August 5,
      2025. https://www.healthline.com/nutrition/6-healthiest-seeds.

231   Pes, Giovanni Mario, Giulia Licheri, Sara Soro, Nunzio Pio Longo, Roberta
      Salis, Giulia Tomassini, Caterina Niolu, Alessandra Errigo, and Maria Pina Dore.
      "Overweight: A Protective Factor against Comorbidity in the Elderly." *International*

Journal of Environmental Research and Public Health 16, no. 19 (2019): 3656. https://doi.org/10.3390/ijerph16193656.

232   Centers for Disease Control and Prevention. "Tips for Healthy Eating for a Healthy Weight." December 28, 2023. https://www.cdc.gov/healthy-weight-growth/healthy-eating/index.html.

233   Olsson, Regan. "5 Things That Happen to Your Body When You Skip Meals." Banner Health, October 2, 2022. https://www.bannerhealth.com/healthcareblog/teach-me/here-is-what-happens-when-you-skip-meals.

234   Spritzler, Franziska. "Does Eating Slowly Help You Lose Weight?" *Healthline*, June 18, 2019. https://www.healthline.com/nutrition/eating-slowly-and-weight-loss.

235   Wolfson, Julia A., and Sara N. Bleich. "Is Cooking at Home Associated with Better Diet Quality or Weight-Loss Intention?" *Public Health Nutrition* 18, no. 8 (2015): 1397–406. https://doi.org/10.1017/S1368980014001943.

236   Mansfield, Rob. "Could You Eat 30 Plant-Based Foods a Week?" World Cancer Research Fund International, September 27, 2021. https://www.wcrf.org/about-us/news-and-blogs/could-you-eat-30-plant-based-foods-each-week/.

237   Spritzler, Franziska. "How Cooking Affects the Nutrient Content of Foods." *Healthline*, November 7, 2019. https://www.healthline.com/nutrition/cooking-nutrient-content.

238   Spritzler, Franziska. "What Is the Healthiest Way to Cook Meat?" *Healthline*, August 13, 2020. https://www.healthline.com/nutrition/healthiest-way-to-cook-meat.

239   Kendrick, Stacey. "Four Heart-Healthy Diet Tips to Add Flavor to Your Food." Vanderbilt Health, April 28, 2023. https://my.vanderbilthealth.com/heart-healthy-diet-tips/.

240   National Cancer Institute. "Chemicals in Meat Cooked at High Temperatures and Cancer Risk." Reviewed July 11, 2017. https://www.cancer.gov/about-cancer/causes-prevention/risk/diet/cooked-meats-fact-sheet.

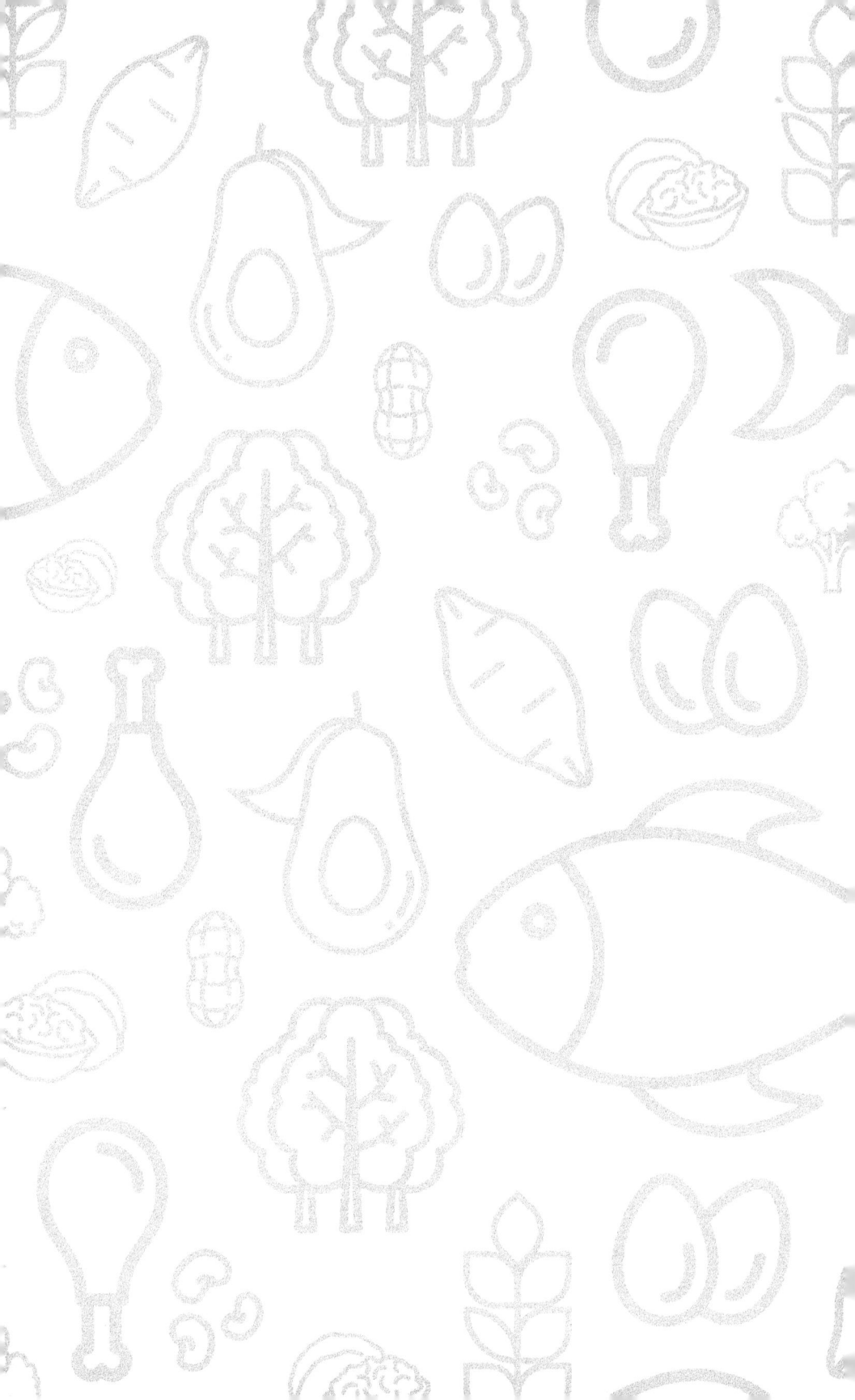

ABOUT THE AUTHOR

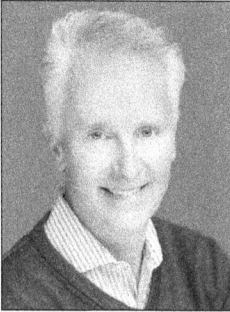

Christopher D. Smith came to the study of diet and nutrition not through formal academic training but through a deep personal motivation. He has experienced several family members passing away early in life from chronic conditions. Many of these health issues are considered preventable and these losses made a lasting impression on him.

As a result, Chris has long been interested in health and wellness. His personal goal has always been to consume a nutritious diet but found that mainstream medical and wellness guidance was often confusing or incomplete. Why was building a healthy diet so confusing? Nutrition, after all, is foundational to long-term health and longevity.

After retiring, Chris resolved to answer that question definitively. Even after reading dozens of articles and multiple scientific studies, he found it surprisingly difficult to assemble a clear picture of what constitutes a fully healthy diet. Determined to solve this puzzle, he turned to the method by which he had always learned best—researching and writing. What began as a personal project grew into a comprehensive effort to evaluate nutrition in a way that was both rigorous and practical.

After over two years of intensive study, Chris discovered that while nutrition is undeniably complex, it *can* be simplified—and translated into an approach that is straightforward, sustainable, and easy to understand. *Absolute Nutrition* presents this framework. He has applied these strategies to his own life with meaningful improvements in energy, physical strength, and overall well-being, and he hopes readers will experience similar benefits.

Born in Richmond, Virginia, Chris spent most of his professional life in Atlanta, Georgia, with several years in Connecticut. He is the father of two grown children and has a close circle of family and friends.

Chris' career was grounded in the insurance industry, culminating in twenty-five years as CEO of a medical malpractice insurance company serving large healthcare systems along the East Coast. His work required close collaboration with respected physicians, hospital leaders, medical school executives, and attorneys. Through this experience, he developed expertise in balancing conflicting priorities, evaluating complex systems, analyzing conflicting information, and distilling intricate issues into clear, actionable strategies.

These same skills proved invaluable in writing *Absolute Nutrition*. His attention to detail, comfort with ambiguity, and patience in navigating incomplete or conflicting data helped him make sense of vast amounts of nutritional research and synthesize it into a coherent, practical approach.

Importantly, Chris has no financial interests tied to the book's recommendations. Every insight in *Absolute Nutrition* is based on independent research and, where evidence was limited, his best reasoned judgment.

His sole purpose in writing this book is to offer readers a clear, usable blueprint for building a truly healthy diet—one that can make a meaningful, positive difference in their lives.